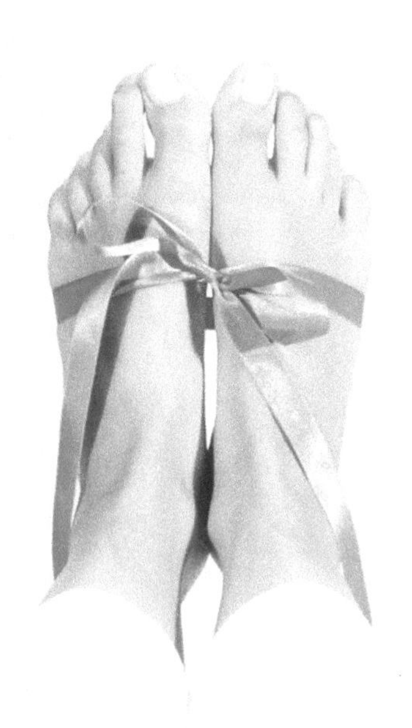

REFLEXOLOGY LYMPH DRAINAGE

ILLUSTRATED **STEP BY STEP GUIDE**
TO THE **SALLY KAY METHOD**

SALLY KAY

Printed in the United Kingdom

Sequence photography by Hamish Kay, Trust Productions Ltd.
(www.trustproductions.co.uk)
Original art work designed and created by Sally Kay®

First Printing, 2019

ISBN: 978-1-9160683-0-8 (Print)
ISBN: 978-1-9160683-1-5 (eBook)

Sally Kay
Rogerstone, Newport
NP10 9LG

www.reflexologylymphdrainage.co.uk

Foreword

It was an honour and privilege to receive a copy of this book. I met Sally, as a visiting academic, whilst she was presenting her innovative work on reflexology and breast cancer. Speed forward five years and I am attending RLD training myself and witnessing award winning Sally sharing her skills and practice worldwide with reflexologists. I now use the technique in my cancer care and hospice work, bringing relief to patients, and I am also finding the approach helpful with others faced with chronic and life limiting diseases.

This book, aside from being a very instructive guide, also provides insights into the theory, development and research work underpinning the RLD package of care. There is detailed guidance in the text given on the process, as well as an excellent overview of lymphoedema, with numerous case studies and supportive literature. Whilst the book is a great stand-alone resource, it is also a "must have" to supplement the face-to-face training and DVD material.

Dr Peter A. Mackereth, PhD, MA, Cert Ed.

Sally Kay's development and articulation of Reflexology Lymph Drainage (RLD) is a must read for both clinicians, healthcare providers and patients. Her development has revolutionised the clinical treatment of not only lymphoedema but lymphatic and vascular disorders (lipoedema, lipolymphoedema, phlebolymphoedema). As a formally trained and certified lymphoedema clinician by the Lymphology Association of North America (CLT-LANA) I treat these types of patients weekly. The reduction in swelling, documented by circumferential measurement (pre and post session) has been drastic and dramatic without failure with RLD whether with or without the standard Manual Lymphatic Drainage (MLD) protocol. I was born with primary lymphoedema (distichiasis) and I have never been able to self-manage (using either or both allopathic and naturopathic techniques) and reduce the swelling in my body over decades of suffering the way that I am now able to with RLD. Finally as a formally trained historian of medicine (PhD), former Research Professor of Public Health, and epidemiologist (MPH), I am awed and privileged to be part of a clinical and medical revolution for a lymphatic treatment that is changing the lives of patients who until now would have to wait much longer for the same outcome.

Dr Sylvia Hood Washington PhD, ND, MPH, MSE, CLT-LANA BCTMB, LMT, RYT-500, HTCP

In a world where conventional medicine is struggling to keep up with the demand for lymphoedema treatments in those surviving cancer, this book comes as a breath of fresh air. It provides the reader with a simple, effective and most importantly, scientifically proven method of treating breast cancer related lymphoedema in a simple non-invasive manner.

Already used by so many reflexologists worldwide, Sally Kay takes you through her RLD journey from beginning to its current end, demonstrating how a simple thought, a lot of work and great support can bring about huge benefits to those experiencing life changing challenges. As a reflexologist, researcher and cancer survivor, I wholeheartedly support the benefits of RLD.

Dr Carol Samuel, PhD, HMAR, FFHT

Disclaimer

Reflexology practice is constantly evolving in response to the needs of those who seek the therapy. It is the responsibility of the reflexologist to maintain professional development and to work within the context of the individual policies and professional guidelines for best practice. The author, other contributors and the publisher are not responsible for any harm or damage to a person, no matter how caused, as a result of information shared in this book.

Contents

Foreword **3**

Disclaimer **5**

Introduction **13**

Section 1: REFLEXOLOGY JOURNEY 15

Chapter 1: My Reflexology Journey **16**
- Inspiration to innovation 28
- My eureka moment! 32

Chapter 2: Small Steps to Research **42**
- Why do we need research? 42
- Simple data collection 44
  - Where do you begin with research? 44
- Developing a conceptual framework 47
  - Here's what happened next 47
- A few highlights 50
- The next step 54

Section 2: FIRST PRINCIPLES OF RLD 59

Chapter 3: The Lymphatic System 60
Lymph 62
Initial lymphatics and lymph vessels 62
Lymph nodes and larger lymph vessels.............................63
Thoracic duct and cisterna chyli 64
Right and left drainage 65
Spleen 65
Other organs of the system 66
Lymph flow 66

Chapter 4: Lymphoedema 68
What is lymphoedema? 68
Primary lymphoedema 68
Secondary lymphoedema 69
Symptoms of lymphoedema 70
Physiological and psychological side effects can include 71
Breast cancer related lymphoedema 72

Chapter 5: Management of Lymphoedema 76
Prevention and self-care 77
Skin care 78
Exercise 79
Compression garments and bandaging 79
Multi-layer lymphoedema bandaging 82
Manual Lymph Drainage (massage) 82
Simple Lymph Drainage exercise 84

Section 3: REFLEXOLOGY LYMPH DRAINAGE 89

Chapter 6: Step by Step Guide to Reflexology Lymph Drainage 90

Introduction 91

Decide where to begin - choose the foot carefully! 93

RLD reflexes - step by step 95

Step 1: The diaphragm 95

Step 2: Spinal cord, cisterna chyli, thoracic duct and subclavian vein 97

Steps 2a & 2b are one move - "down, up & in" 104

Step 3: Cervical lymph nodes, Upper trapezius 105

Summary of 3a & 3b as one move 109

Step 4: Upper lymph reflexes (dorsal) 110

Step 5: Upper lymph to lateral shoulder reflex - deltoid muscle 114

Step 6: Upper lymph to underarm (pump) - Axillary lymph nodes 118

Step 7: Lower lymph 122

Summary of steps 7a & 7b as one move 127

Step 8: Breast reflex 128

Step 9: Arm 131

Step 10: Spleen reflex (left foot only) 136

Step 11: Kidney to bladder flush 137

Step 12: Linking 138

Summary of RLD for unilateral secondary lymphoedema of the arm 139

Summary of RLD reflexes 140

RLD hand reflexes 142

Home help tip 142

Integrating RLD 143

RLD & lymphoedema swelling of the legs 144

RLD & bilateral secondary lymphoedema of the arms 144

RLD & primary lymphoedema and lipoedema 145

RLD & inflammatory and auto-immune conditions 145

Chapter 7: Clinical Reasoning and Best Practice **148**
Contra-indications for RLD 152

Section 4: SPEAKING VOLUMES 155

Chapter 8: Limb Volume Circumference Measurements **156**
How to measure the arm 159
Step by step guide to accurate measurement 161
How to convert the circumference measurements into volume 163

Chapter 9: Data and Research **167**
Participant 1 168
Participant 2 170
Participant 3 172
Participant 4 174
Participant 5 176
Participant 6 178
RLD research abstract 1 180
RLD research abstract 2 182
RLD research abstract 3 183

Section 5: THE RIPPLE EFFECT 185

Chapter 10: RLD Case Studies and Testimonials **186**
Case studies 188
Case study 1: Breast cancer related lymphoedema 188
Case study 2: Palliative 192
Case study 3: Secondary lymphoedema, post-operative inflammation and pain 194
Case study 4: Bartholin's cyst 196
Case study 5: Breast cancer related lymphoedema of the arm 198
Case study 6: Psoriatic arthritis 199

Case study 7: Lower limb swelling ... 201
Case study 8: Breast cancer related lymphoedema ... 205
Case study 9: Breast cancer related lymphoedema ... 207
Testimonials from reflexologists and clients ... 209
1. Gail Davies ... 209
2. Jan Rose, reflexologist - suitcase to clutch bag! ... 211
3. Ethne, research participant ... 212
4. Reflexologist Rachael Posner's case study ... 213
5. Dorothy Lawrie - primary lymphoedema ... 213

Chapter 11: The Full Circle ... 216
Back to the roots of reflexology ... 216

Chapter 12: The Future ... 221
Making waves with the ripple effect ... 221

Appendices ... 225

Step this way ... 226

Useful sources of information ... 227
Books ... 227
Websites ... 228

Glossary ... 230

Image Index ... 232
Charts ... 232
Images ... 233
Tables ... 234

Index ... 235

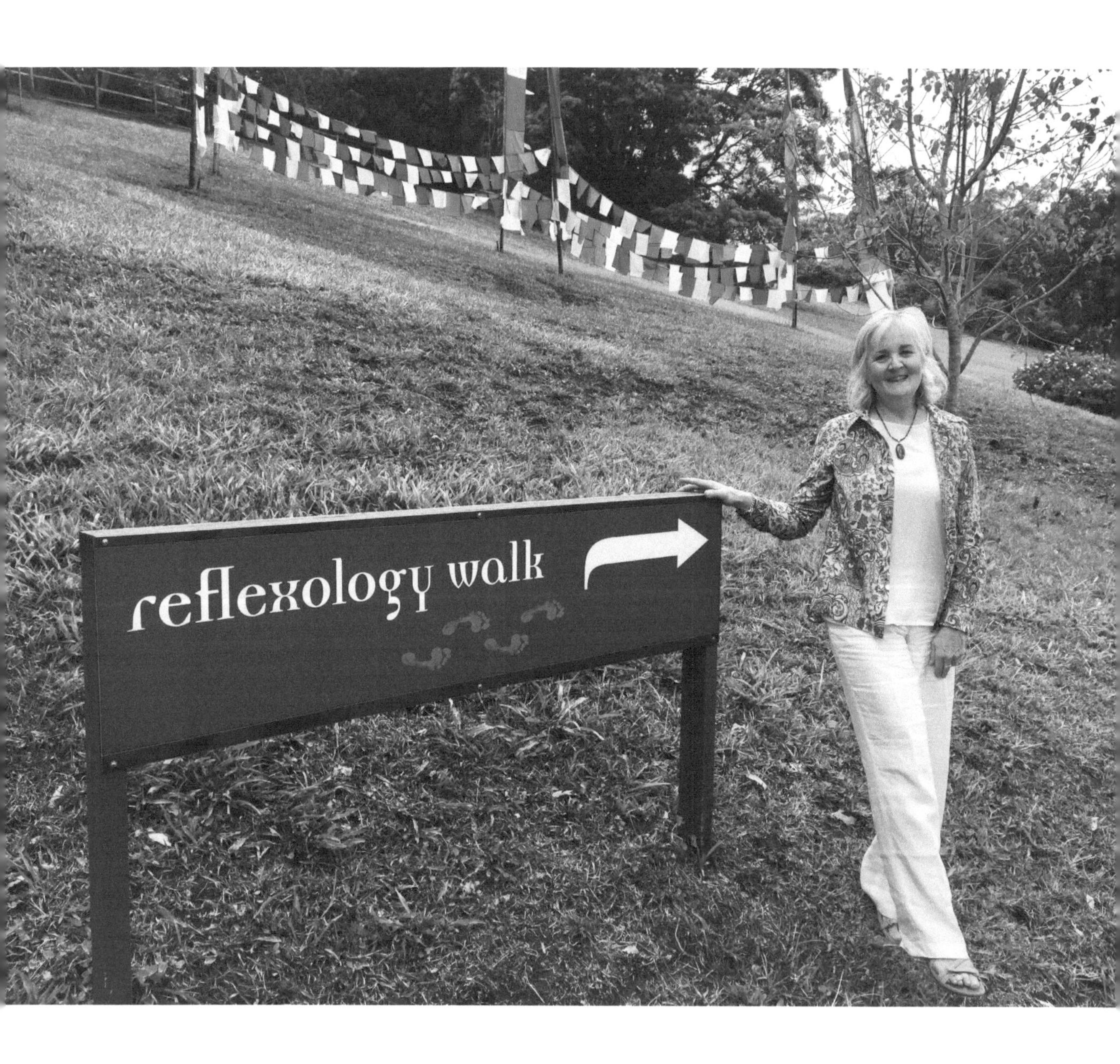
reflexology walk

Introduction

This book is a labour of love about my reflexology journey and the creation of Reflexology Lymph Drainage (RLD). You will learn about the first principles of RLD and how the desire to help patients with breast cancer related lymphoedema inspired me to research and develop the original treatment protocol. For this innovation to be successful I had to think outside the box and forge my own pathway. As a result, I figured out how to isolate the reflexes of the lymphatic system on the feet and work in a methodical order to cause a beneficial effect on the body.

This approach has delivered consistent, phenomenal results. The facts and figures underline the impact my method of RLD has when these techniques are applied. There is such a positive ripple effect on quality of life when the swelling diminishes and lost self-confidence returns. To many people it is a gift of hope in a previously hopeless situation.

From my clinical experience I knew RLD was working and being able to measure the results is an exciting prospect for us all. You will find out in this book what happened when I took a few small steps towards research. See the ripple effect and the results of the studies which followed.

Learn why RLD flows sequentially, and how each reflex has a role in stimulating the drainage function. Discover how to map these reflexes on the feet (and hands) using the anatomical reflection theory of reflexology and understand the relationship of each. For this purpose, I have included a simple review of the lymphatic system that explains why RLD moves in a defined, logical sequence to achieve these potentially life changing results.

Follow the beautifully illustrated step by step guide for reflexologists to implement the RLD protocol laid out in this book. It can be used as a stand-alone treatment, and ultimately it provides a simple and effective tool for the reflexology tool box, one that is easy to integrate into your everyday practice.

Learn how reflexology treatment enables tangible and intangible outcomes to be measured, and why data collection and analysis is beneficial to our profession. Consider the value in the eyes of other healthcare providers and importantly, those who are responsible for the allocation of future healthcare funding.

Bridging the gap between reflexology practice and proving its worth is notoriously difficult. I hope that my initial RLD research project may form the cornerstone of future studies which will contribute to the understanding and integration of reflexology. By working together in a consistent manner to build a compelling body of evidence, I believe we can continue to expand the credibility and reach of our profession together.

"Human behaviour flows from three main sources: desire, emotion, and knowledge." - Plato

The creation of RLD came from the desire to help relieve the physical and emotional symptoms of lymphoedema, with knowledge of the lymphatic system and Manual Lymph Drainage. I learnt to question things rather than to just ask questions.

I invite reflexologists all over the world to join me on this remarkable reflexology journey, and this book shows you how you can be part of it.

Section 1

REFLEXOLOGY JOURNEY

Chapter 1
My Reflexology Journey

Reflexology serendipitously found me when I needed it most, and like a magic carpet it picked me up before I hit rock bottom. Since then this magic carpet has truly taken off, at times with me hanging on to the fringes for dear life. As it continues to gain momentum I am learning to avoid resistance, and to enjoy the ride and just go with it.

I was introduced to reflexology in 2004 by a family member who was a big fan of complementary therapies. During a very stressful time, she invited me for a session with a reflexologist that she used to see every few weeks, to help me cope with everything I was going through. I was absolutely amazed at how much better I felt by the end of the reflexology treatment. I felt "normal" again, and all the stress and pressure had lifted. I felt lighter, which was a strange and unfamiliar feeling, a peaceful respite from stress and anxiety. My head was clear and my stomach was no longer tied up in knots. I felt so relaxed and it was the first time I had felt this way in a very long time.

This first experience of reflexology was like being thrown a lifeline and it was crystal clear to me that I needed to find out more about it. Within a few months I enrolled at the local further education college on a holistic therapy course, which included reflexology.

Since then I have realised that most reflexologists find their way into the profession through personal experience of the therapeutic effects and benefits. You never forget that first positive reflexology session and to this day I completely understand when people say that they feel "normal" and "lighter", whether it's physically or emotionally. It's all good!

Initially I was only interested in the reflexology course, but this was part time and expensive. Luckily the full-time course was free to adult learners in Wales and it included reflexology. I shall always be grateful for the opportunity that funded adult education in Wales gave to me.

The syllabus included several modules: massage, aromatherapy, reflexology, anatomy and physiology, health and safety. It was just the beginning of an enlightening and inspiring journey into the world of complementary therapies.

Thanks to the course tutor Ted Kelland, who had a wonderful ability to inspire learners, I became truly engaged in education for the first time in my life, albeit late - in my mid-forties - but it was the right time for me and I loved every second of it.

Much of Ted's philosophy came from life experience. He had the ability to put things in perspective with anecdotal stories to make them relevant. Strange though it may seem for a lecturer in complementary therapies, his previous career was as a Royal Marine Commando in the special forces spanning 25 years. Much of his time in the military was spent overseas where he first developed an interest in complementary and alternative medicine (CAM). Amongst other things he had studied Chinese medicine, acupuncture, herbal and energy medicine and reflexology in China, crystal therapy in Hawaii and was also a master of seven different martial arts.

Tuition for theory and bodywork classes went above and beyond the syllabus, and the standard learning objectives for certification with the awarding body. Instead of a box ticking exercise, for example learning to identify the bones of the skeletal system by labelling a picture, he required a 2000-word essay about the structure and function for each system of the body, and insisted on Harvard referencing. Years later, I was grateful for his gentle introduction to academia.

Ted was on a mission to inspire learners. It was engaging and interesting and I was totally captivated, completely absorbed and inspired. So much can be achieved with praise and the right encouragement. Although I decided to concentrate on reflexology it was some time later that I really appreciated the true value of the width of my learning.

As with many of these complementary therapies there is often an overlap between modalities: similarities which date back thousands of years. Reflexology is widely believed to have roots in ancient cultures, Egyptian, Chinese, Greek, Indian and Roman, so where did it all begin? Surely there must be something in it for so many of the ancient civilisations to lay claim to it.

The historical holistic approach to wellbeing championed by Ted is based on the idea that reflexology and other complementary therapies are used to stay well rather than to fix when things go wrong.

In 2016 I was lucky enough to be invited to visit China, surely the ultimate destination for a reflexologist! This gave me the chance to compare and contrast my approach against techniques that have changed little for thousands of years (see Chapter 11 on page 216).

There is a distinct lack of scientific research that proves conclusively that reflexology works, but on the other hand there is not much to prove it does not work either!

The single most important lesson I learnt from Ted was to question things and to become a free thinker. I learnt not to accept all that we hear or are taught, but instead to pause for a moment and ask, "Why?" If the answer is "Just because it is" or "THEY said" - well then ask, "Who are THEY?" and "How do THEY know?"

The learning outcomes of the course required things to be done in a certain way, which he taught. While best practice in reflexology training is often questionable and subject to much discussion and debate, we all have to start somewhere and the learning objectives need to be met. These vary greatly and depend very much on the syllabus of the awarding body, the approach and life experiences of the tutor, different foot maps and of course personal experience and interpretation of all of this.

There are many grey areas in complementary therapies, treatment outcomes that we cannot explain and plenty of mystifying questions and inexplicable answers. In my opinion, the real learning begins once we have qualified and start practising, putting our new skills to the test, and in doing so we never stop learning.

Learning the basics of any discipline is essential and the lectures were full of interesting facts as well as anecdotal evidence, but then they would often finish with, "Ah but, is it the intention? Who knows?"

Every time a new foot map is developed it needs to be different from others to avoid copyright issues. Yet in spite of these perceived differences in reflex areas, it is not possible to be absolutely sure where any of the reflexes are on any foot map. It is an interesting exercise to trace several different foot maps and lay one on top of another to compare and contrast, a way to extract ideas for new innovative techniques, then trial them for effectiveness. It leaves me with more questions than answers!

Until we fully understand the mechanism of action for the likes of reflexology, it will remain firmly rooted in multiple different theories and beliefs. In the meantime it is good to question things, to implement new but well considered approaches and to justify our reasons for choices when working in a particular way.

For me, a foot map is merely for guidance and as a reference when training to become a reflexologist. In practice, people's bodies are different shapes and sizes, as are their feet. Therefore, I prefer a three dimensional approach and an anatomical reflection theory. For example, to stimulate the spinal reflexes, feel and look for the bones on the feet. For soft tissue like the buttocks which provide protective padding around the pelvis, reflexes are the soft pad of the heel. Bone for bone and soft tissue for soft tissue (see Fig. 01).

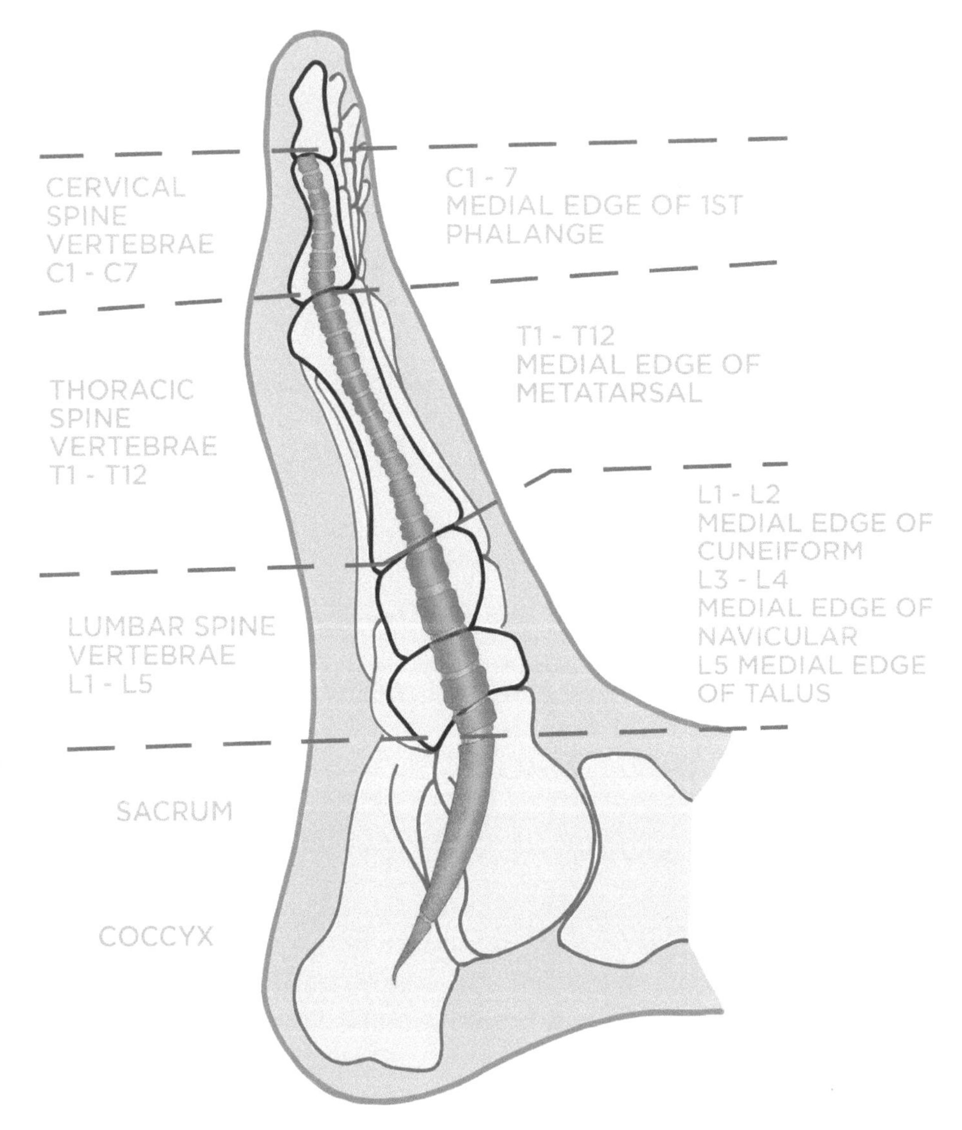

Fig. 01: Anatomical reference for spine reflexes

Pertinence and logic helped to inspire me with the clinical application of Reflexology Lymph Drainage (RLD), and the subsequent research and development. It was this fundamental principle of questioning things, rather than just accepting all that we are told. In trying to comprehend the bigger therapeutic picture of reflexology, its methods, history, beliefs, foot maps, efficacy and ultimately the mechanism of action. What would happen if the lymphatic system reflexes on the feet were isolated and worked in a way to mirror Manual Lymph Drainage? There is so much to consider.

After this first course, I was hungry for more knowledge and a greater understanding, as it had left me with so many unanswered questions. A case of the more I learn, the less I know, which continues to this day. The experience of giving and receiving treatments, as well as all the case study work and reflective practice during the training, was a revelation. It was the beginning of a journey of personal development, enlightenment and freedom from many self-limiting beliefs.

In 2005, as a newly qualified holistic therapist, I did what many new graduates do and enrolled on a series of other continuing professional development (CPD) courses. I became a CPD junkie! These included Indian head massage, crystal therapy, thermo-auricular therapy, hot-stone massage and reiki. In spite of all of these additional skills, my passion still lay with reflexology. There was no getting away from it.

Slowly and surely, after qualifying I began to build up a small private practice. Attracting clients can be the biggest challenge to a newly qualified therapist. In the early years, I tried all sorts of marketing strategies without ever paying for advertising. I designed, printed and delivered thousands of local flyers, with approximately less than 1% response rate. There was a local Natural Health Show, where I had a stand with a colleague and here we provided endless taster sessions of reflexology. In my experience, word of mouth is the best form of marketing and it only takes a few regular clients and satisfied customers to start spreading the word and soon the client base begins to grow. This proactive approach to marketing involved giving talks to local businesses, networking groups, schools, women's groups, the WI, charities and support groups, something I really enjoy doing to this day.

A year later, in 2006, through a chance meeting with another therapist at one of these CPD courses, I first learnt about Hospice of the Valleys, and within a few months was offered a position working there part time as one of a team of complementary therapists.

Hospice of the Valleys is a charity based in the South Wales Valleys, founded in 1991 by Dr Richard Lamerton, who had a vision for future cancer care in Blaenau Gwent. He was inspired after working alongside Dame Cicely Saunders (1918–2005), a leading figure in the campaign to establish hospices around the world. She is credited with being the founder of the modern hospice movement, with an international reputation for influencing thinking about death in many countries. Dame Cicely believed that the final days of a person's life could be made happy, and she helped to change society's attitude towards end of life and dying.

> **"You matter because you are you, and you matter to the last moment of your life."** – Dame Cicely Saunders

At the time, Hospice of the Valleys was a hospice without walls and did not have its own premises, only rented office space. The medical team saw patients in their own homes as well as at a number of satellite drop-in clinics, where patients and their carers could attend for help and support. These clinics were informal and provided a very caring, nurturing and holistic environment for all service users. They were run by specialist nurses, with the support of social workers, complementary therapists and volunteer hosts, hostesses and drivers, who looked after everyone. There was always a warm Welsh welcome and a plentiful supply of tea, coffee and homemade cakes.

Four times a week, half-day clinics were held in a variety of makeshift venues across different areas of the south-east Wales valleys. These included a rugby club, a choir hall, a working men's club, a chapel and a community centre. Complementary therapies were available to both patients and their carers, and no appointment was necessary. It was all very flexible and if anyone arrived feeling particularly distressed or unwell they were seen immediately and given extra treatment time if it was needed.

Complementary therapies available at these makeshift drop-in clinics included reflexology, massage, aromatherapy, Manual Lymph Drainage massage (MLD), reiki, and Indian head massage from a small team of therapists at each clinic. Group work was also offered at some of the clinics, and small groups worked together doing visualisation and meditation as well as learning Simple Lymph Drainage (SLD), a gentle self-help exercise. This was taught to patients who had been diagnosed with secondary lymphoedema, or to those who were at risk of developing it.

Once lymph nodes have been removed there is a lifetime risk of developing lymphoedema swelling. In some cases it happens soon after surgery, others may not get it for years, and some will not develop it at all.

Being part of this supportive multi-disciplined team was a privilege. Witnessing first-hand how complementary therapies were being used to make a real difference to the quality of people's lives, and deaths, made it very rewarding work. The simple things, such as women being once again able to wear their wedding ring at end of life, should not be underestimated in their importance.

> An important part of a therapist's training is learning about and understanding the risks of cautions and contra-indications to ensure patient safety and best practice. It can be challenging to work with clients and patients who have such complex medical history, conditions, side effects of medication, surgery, chemotherapy, radiotherapy and the psychological impact of a cancer diagnosis, or any life limiting condition.

The working environment at Hospice of the Valleys was supportive of both staff and service users, with the specialist nurses and an experienced team of multi-disciplined therapists. Help and support was always available. In my experience, this outstanding level of peer support and supervision is vital for anyone providing therapies in hospice care and helps immensely to sustain a healthy work-life balance and self-care.

Twice a month Hospice of the Valleys held a clinic on a Saturday. This was by appointment only and patients stayed for a whole day of relaxation and support. There was a choice of therapies, with plenty of time for each session of massage, reflexology, aromatherapy, reiki, counselling, and art therapy. There were gentle yoga and meditation classes, as well as tai chi and chi kung, teaching basic self-help strategies. For example, a simple yoga breathing exercise can be used to help manage anxiety by re-focusing the attention on the breathing. It has a calming effect and can be used anytime or anywhere.

Not all service users accessed the complementary therapy services. Instead some of the patients came just to see the nurse or social worker and others appreciated the social and community support of others.

Complementary therapies were used to support patients and help them through each stage of the disease, from diagnosis to discharge, or to end of life care. Domiciliary visits were also available for patients who were not well enough to attend the clinic. Providing a home visit was a very different therapeutic experience for both the patient and therapist, compared to working at the clinics. Extra care is taken for the comfort of the patient, who is likely to be less mobile, and means the therapy needs to be adapted accordingly for comfort and support of the individual. A gentle reflexology treatment can be given through the hands if feet are inaccessible or they are too swollen. No matter how the reflexology treatment differs in terms of pressure or specific techniques, in my experience it is always well received.

I noticed sometimes how the positive effect of the treatment on the patient was also felt by the family. The ripple effect of seeing a loved one enjoy a nurturing therapeutic experience is comforting for the whole family.

After the first year working at the hospice, I had learnt so much from both patients and colleagues. Providing therapies for 20-30 people a week is a lot of feet! It's true that it is only after we qualify that the learning really begins! Each week through the clinical experience of working with the presenting concerns of all service users, patients and their carers, it was obvious to me just how much people benefitted from receiving these treatments.

Most of these cases were complex and may be considered as "text book contra-indications" to complementary therapies. I learnt so much about how therapies could be adapted safely to help and support those who needed it most, from the positive responses of the patients and service users along with the support from experienced colleagues, who were generous in sharing their knowledge.

Knowledge, information and understanding is the key to safe practice. It helps when making an informed choice on how best to adapt reflexology (or any complementary therapy) when people present with a complex medical history, symptoms of ongoing health conditions and the side effects of medication. Knowledge of anatomy and physiology and the pathology of a condition, processes of the disease, information about the effect of medical treatments, side effects and symptoms - all of these help to understand how best to proceed safely.

For the newly qualified reflexologist, understanding the pathology of the disease helps with adapting the treatment protocol safely when working with this patient group while being mindful of the cautions and contra-indications.

This invaluable clinical experience clearly demonstrated to me just how much comfort reflexology (and other therapies) provide through the relaxing effects of these treatments which are more accepted in palliative care these days. With the chronic stress, tension and high levels of anxiety which are often associated with a cancer diagnosis and treatment, reflexology is a great way to press the reset button. It helps people to cope and feel better about themselves as they come to terms with a diagnosis and everything else they are going through. Even if it does only provide a brief period of respite, the relaxation and a calmer mindset can help in an immeasurable way. After all, it is not possible for the body to be in the stressed state, "fight-and-flight" at the same time as a relaxed, "heal-and-grow" (or "rest-and-digest") one. It is so much more than just a placebo, as is believed by some.

As well as relaxation, reflexology seemed to bring about some welcome relief from many of the physical symptoms and side effects of treatments and medications that patients had, for example, constipation, sleeplessness, nausea and pain. Something was definitely happening and I needed to know more!

While Hospice of the Valleys provided a nurturing environment to work in, even with the support of the team, my quest for greater understanding, broader knowledge and further insight into the application of reflexology and the mechanism of action was a driving force to learn more! So in 2007, with encouragement from my family, I enrolled on the BSc (Hons) in Complementary Therapies at the University of Wales Institute Cardiff (UWIC, now Cardiff Metropolitan University). Going to university and studying for a degree was something I could not have imagined myself ever doing, not even in my wildest dreams. I had taken the next step - onwards and upwards!

I chose to study part time over four years instead of full time over three, so that I could carry on working at Hospice of the Valleys and by this time I also had a small private practice of loyal clientele.

Tragically at the end of my first year at university, Ted Kelland passed away after a short illness. Ironically it was a few months after he had received the Welsh Inspirational Tutor of the Year award. Inspired by Ted, I will continue to champion reflexology and RLD research, development, education and sharing with others. He is sadly missed by those who knew him, his fellow "eagles". One of his favourite sayings was, "It's hard to soar like an eagle, when you're surrounded by turkeys". His words not mine, but I get his meaning and the sentiment stays with me.

The second year of my degree included the reflexology bodywork module, taught by Judith Whatley. In the very first lecture, she said that magic word, "Why?" She had asked the all-important question, and I knew it was going to be a good year! In fact, it was the beginning of a friendship, mutual respect and a shared passion for reflexology and collaboration on further research into RLD. Working together we are stronger, able to maximise our collective strengths through sharing and collaboration.

At the end of this academic year I was lucky enough to spend two months working as the residential massage therapist at the internationally acclaimed holistic holiday retreat, Atsitsa Bay, on the Greek island of Skyros. The year before, I had met a young patient at one of the clinics who went there for a holiday, and came back two weeks later like a new woman. Her transformation was truly remarkable. I needed to find out more about this place, and duly sent for a brochure. When it arrived, at the bottom of the page it said, "therapies payable for separately on site". I wrote them a letter, and was thrilled to be offered the position for the following season. The timing was perfect after two years at university with another two to go. I needed a break.

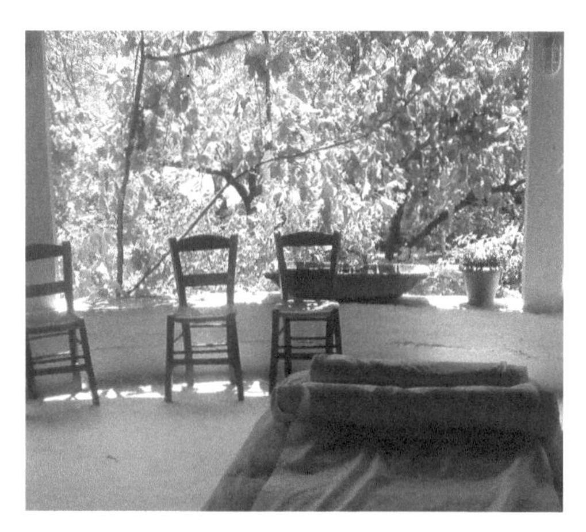

Fig. 02: Atsitsa, August 2009

Time spent in Atsitsa provides opportunities to try new things, in a fun and held space, a place where anything is possible. A chance to step out of your comfort zone, to expand your mind, body and spirit is a life affirming experience, one that I am truly grateful for. Like an elastic band that gets well and truly stretched, it never quite returns to its original state. It has become one of my favourite holiday destinations. Always a magic place to be and each visit is a unique experience.

Five years of working at the hospice was such a privilege, and a wonderful learning experience. It was a real opportunity to put the gift of reflexology to incredibly good use. The clinical practice of giving between 20 and 30 treatments a week gave me invaluable clinical experience, in parallel with the in-depth studying for the degree. The majority of these treatments were reflexology. The more I used it the more convinced I became of its efficacy. I just needed to find a way of validating this belief.

Inspiration to innovation

My passion for reflexology continued to grow and the clinical experience supported my belief in the therapeutic possibilities. This provided me with the confidence to think outside the box.

Sessions at the drop-in clinics were time limited. It was not possible to do a full reflexology treatment unless you rushed through all the reflexes, which I find unsatisfactory. Instead of doing this, mine was a different approach. Treatment always depended on how the patient was on the day. I would respectfully ask about their main concerns, before deciding how best to give an adaptive shorter reflexology treatment which was always tailored accordingly to best meet their needs and ensure safe practice.

This time-limited, problem-specific reflexology treatment usually starts by gently working the diaphragm reflex, nervous system and spinal cord reflexes before focusing on a more problem-specific area or system of the body.

The patient's main concerns were often related to the side effects from a cocktail of medications. A common complaint, for example, would be constipation, a recognised and well documented known side effect of some of the painkiller medication. As reflexologists, it is widely accepted that reflexology can help the body with digestion and elimination imbalances.

A reflexology treatment plan for patients with this unwelcome side effect of constipation would focus on all the digestion and elimination reflexes, after working the diaphragm and spinal cord reflexes. The rationale behind it was that by working the diaphragm reflex, all ten zones of the body were covered and the nervous system and spinal cord would reach everything else before tailoring the rest to a more specific problem.

I believe we should always work anatomically and in harmony with the body, stimulating the colon reflex in a clockwise direction to support the elimination and function of the digestive system. Work the large intestine reflexes clockwise from the ascending colon, to the transverse colon, then the descending colon into the Sigmoid colon. Many of the patients who received this adaptive approach to reflexology treatments reported positive benefits, often immediately!

The more this happened the more I adapted my approach to all reflexology treatment for many other presenting problems and side effects often seen in the clinics. As previously mentioned I believe it is good practice to understand the underlying causes for presenting conditions and modify each session to the individual.

The realisation that it is possible to give an effective targeted reflexology treatment without working all the reflexes for every system of the body was a light bulb moment. Reflexology really does work!

In the case of someone with a headache presenting for reflexology, it could be due to any number of underlying causes, which might include anything from stress, tension and anxiety to something more physical or serious. A reflexology treatment plan for a stress related tension headache would start with reflexes for the diaphragm and spinal cord (central nervous system) and then focus on the neck and shoulder reflexes. A relaxing sequence could be carried out to help relieve the tension and thus ease the headache. Likewise, if the cause is sinus congestion the sinus and lymphatic reflexes would be included. The benefits became very apparent to me, reinforcing my belief that RLD was potentially a useful innovation.

Working this way was proving to be an extremely effective method. At the clinics many of the patients suffered with secondary lymphoedema following treatment for breast cancer. The hospice therapist who provided Manual Lymph Drainage massage (MLD) as well as the Simple Lymph Drainage (SLD) self-help exercises was off sick for a prolonged period, due to a fall, and was unable to work. During this time patients frequently asked, "I don't suppose you could do anything for my arm could you? It's been aching." Although I have body massage and advanced massage qualifications, I am not a qualified MLD practitioner. MLD is a specialist type of massage (see Chapter 5 on page 76).

With clinical experience, a good knowledge of massage and an understanding of the lymphatic system, it occurred to me that maybe if I could isolate the lymphatic reflexes on the feet, and work them in a sequence that would mirror the principle of MLD and SLD, it might just cause an effect on the lymphatic system. In the same way, a treatment focused on the digestion and elimination reflexes seemed to cause an immediate effect on the bowels. Instinctively I had begun to put the theory of reflexology to the test.

With the full permission of each patient who presented with secondary lymphoedema, I started to explore the idea of isolating the reflexes of the lymphatic system. The intention being that this would cause an effect on the drainage function and reduce the lymphoedema swelling in the arm. The focus of this early RLD reflexology treatment was entirely on the lymphatic reflexes, whilst paying close attention to verbal feedback and the physiological responses to the treatment.

> The sequence of RLD is based on the anatomy, physiology and function of the lymphatic system, and the principles of Manual Lymph Drainage massage (MLD) and Simple Lymph Drainage exercises (SLD). RLD uses the reflexology anatomical reflection theory to mirror these principles on the corresponding reflexes of the feet.

Patients likened the sensations they experienced during this newly adapted reflexology to those felt during MLD, entirely without the power of suggestion. I had no idea what they might feel during these sessions. Some of these sensations included very light pins and needles, tingling, light feathering, fluttering, a ripple, a wave, flow and movement in the arms. There were reported changes in urination, increased volume and urgency, as well as reports of stronger darker urine. Something was definitely happening!

Less is more with the power of suggestion and to this day still something I avoid when it comes to what may be felt during any reflexology treatment. If asked, "What will I feel during the treatment?", my usual vague answer is, "Everybody is different." By keeping it vague we avoid the power of suggestion and in doing so any feedback is authentic. In reverse if you tell a client what they might feel and they experience nothing, they are less likely to accept the reflexology has done anything for them. Instead they risk becoming someone who says, "Tried that once and it didn't work, it did nothing for me."

As the weeks passed and more and more of the patients heard about the perceived effects, they too wanted to try this adapted reflexology for their lymphoedema after seeing the results others were experiencing. The results seemed to be almost instantaneous, and the effects, which included visibly looser clothing and jewellery, improved range of movement of the shoulder and less discomfort and pain. Patients also reported the results were lasting from one week to the next. Some found they could wear clothes they had not been able to wear for months, sometimes years, because they had become too tight in the arm. The results were truly astounding.

By now it was June 2010 and I was busy preparing for my final year of the degree, and the dissertation. The research proposal assignment had been submitted and I was all set to carry out a survey about the use of complementary therapies in supportive cancer care. I wasn't excited by the prospect of it, merely going through the motions.

My eureka moment!

While working I continued to explore and develop this adapted approach to reflexology for the patients with lymphoedema, tailoring it to each patient individually. The results appeared to be consistently quite incredible, and patients reported lasting benefits from one week to the next after receiving this treatment. Then one day at the clinic, I used a tape measure to take a couple of circumferential measurements around a patient's swollen arm before and after this adapted treatment was given.

The proximal section of the arm was where most of the swelling was visible. These measurements were not taken scientifically and therefore were not particularly accurate, but nevertheless there appeared to be an instant reduction of more than 1cm to the upper arm. The results were undeniable, far exceeding my expectations, but there it was! By coincidence a new palliative care consultant had just started working for the hospice and was present as an observer in the clinic that day.

It was a **eureka** moment, something that I will always remember. I knew then that I had to take this forward, no matter what hurdles lay ahead. I was beside myself with excitement at the prospect of an objective measurable result to show the effect of a reflexology treatment. I rushed home, changed and drove straight to the university to speak to Judith about it and the possibility of changing my final year research proposal which had already been submitted.

It had to be done even though it would involve a lot more work. For a start, a new research proposal had to be written. It was worth it, and that summer was spent preparing all the documentation and re-writing the research proposal. This was submitted to both the university and the hospice clinical governance committee. They supported the proposal but conducting clinical research on hospice patients meant that NHS ethical approval was required for the study. This was a giant hurdle but also another challenge I was relishing. Looking back I'm not sure how I managed it.

From the early days of the degree and the very first "introduction to research" module, it was made clear that final year research projects would not be possible if NHS ethical approval was required. The application process was an unknown quantity, and none of the previous graduates had been in this position. Eventually it was agreed that I could try it at my own risk, but I was warned this would involve a lot of extra work, and indeed it did. There were no guarantees the application would be successful and there was a risk of not being able to graduate if it was a lengthy process. Undeterred, I continued with the application, which was probably even more work than the actual final dissertation. It was a challenging and arduous process.

The ethics committee has to ensure safe practice and that no harm would be done. As part of the submission, a detailed account of the proposed intervention was required, in this case the Reflexology Lymph Drainage (RLD) treatment protocol. This is when RLD was first formalised, because each participant has to receive the same intervention and the ethics committee needed to understand exactly what this would involve and what the risk factors were.

In the meantime the clinical services director at the hospice arranged training for me in the standardised method of Limb Volume Circumference Measurements (LVCM), commonly used by the lymphoedema service at that time. The volume of the arm is treated like a cylinder, and both arms are measured in order to calculate the difference between the swollen arm and the contralateral normal arm. The volume of the normal arm is subtracted from the volume of the swollen arm, and the difference is the excess swelling (see How to measure the arm on page 159).

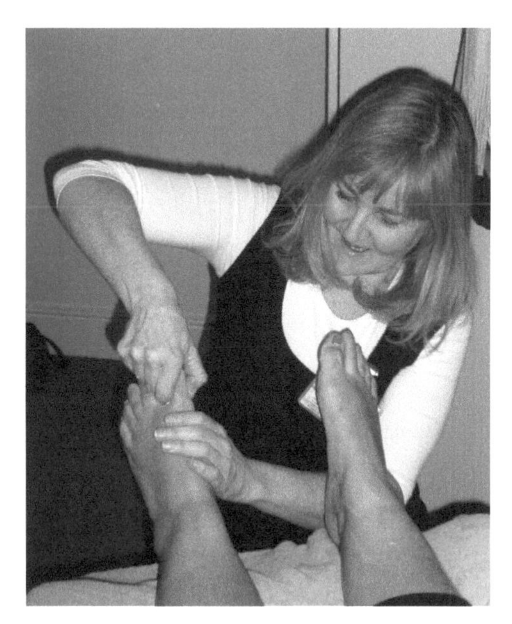

Fig. 03: Hospice of the Valleys, February 2011

Thankfully I had the support and encouragement of the palliative care consultant who was present in the clinic that day, and he kindly helped me to register and start the online application for NHS ethics approval. As with many things, that first step is the hardest and once I got into it, I just waded through, taking lots of small steps, a bit at a time.

Once all the documentation for the NHS ethics application had been accepted, applicants are invited to attend a meeting with the regional ethics committee. In this case the committee was a panel of 12 people including consultants, nurses and lay people. All of the committee members received a hard copy of the application. The meeting was an opportunity to clarify and discuss any relevant questions or concerns they may have had about the proposal with the researcher. Quite an ordeal for a sole practitioner!

After careful consideration, the NHS research ethics committee approved the application subject to a couple of minor amendments. In January 2011 six participants were recruited into the study, which took six weeks to complete (see Chapter 2 on page 42 and Chapter 9 on page 167).

Later that year I graduated with a First Class Honours degree in Complementary Therapies and a prize for the best dissertation. Graduation day was one of the proudest moments of my life.

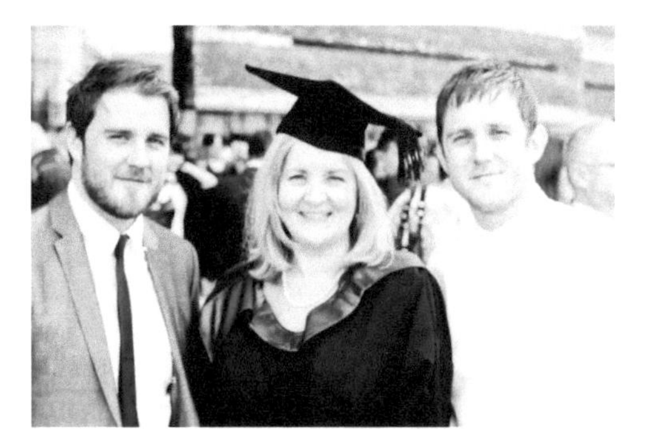

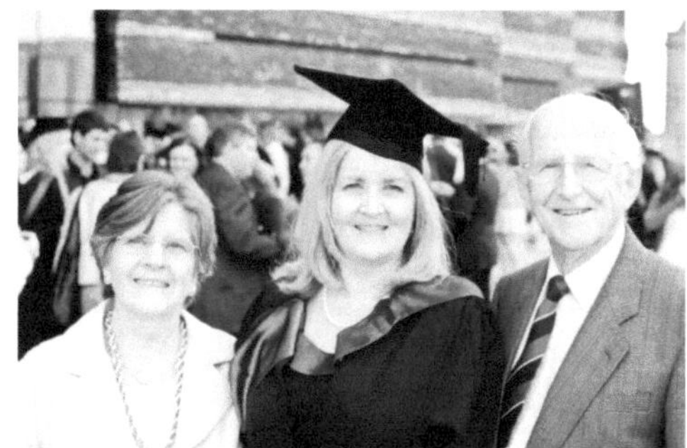

Fig. 04: **My graduation, July 2011**

Coinciding with the end of the degree, the job at Hospice of the Valleys came to a natural end as they wanted to employ a full-time therapist instead of a part-time team.

Still needing regular part-time work to supplement the ebb and flow of private practice, I got a job as a therapist at the local cancer hospital one day a week. Initially I was delighted and excited to work within the health service, naively assuming it would be like working for Hospice of the Valleys, but sadly that was not the case.

I found the lack of flexibility and pressure to conform too stifling and nonsensical "rules" meant I felt unable to do my best for the patients. I also missed the peer support and supervision available at the hospice. Sadly, in hindsight, this was a wrong turn on my RLD journey and another difficult time. Stressed by the working environment and worried about how I could afford to carry on working as a therapist, I came close to giving up and even applied for a job in a bra shop!

As the stress and frustration took its toll on me, in 2012 I developed alopecia. In March that year, with my hair loss at its worst, I presented the results of my undergraduate study as an abstract poster presentation at the Complementary and Alternative Medicine Strategy for Research and Development (CAMSTRAND) research conference, with the bald patches on my head lightly coloured with three different eyebrow pencils, a useful tip I read online for alopecia sufferers. Thankfully this presentation was very well received.

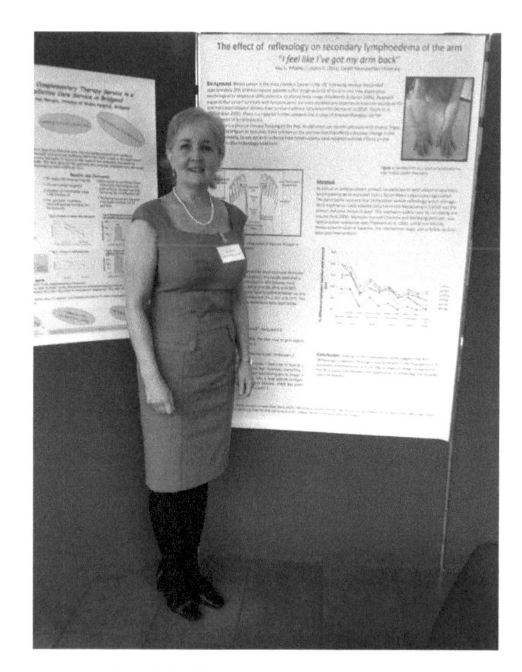

Fig. 05: Poster presentation at CAMSTRAND, 29th March 2012

Delegates at the CAMSTRAND conference included leading CAM

academics who were interested in the research, as well as other reflexology practitioners. Gradually people began to enquire about RLD, asking if training was available. With that another door opened and all that hard work wasn't going to be wasted after all.

Around the time, Judith's words were, "There's a PhD here!" We discussed at length the possibility of doing further academic research and ultimately a doctorate, but after four years of studying for the degree I decided to embark on a more practical path than the academic route. From that moment on I became a woman on a mission, full of drive and determination!

This was another pivotal moment in the life of RLD, the research, training courses and ultimately writing this book. It's a labour of love that's been a long time coming.

Choosing this more practical route meant a greater number of people would have access to RLD within a shorter time frame. I focused all my attention on this and began to spread the word. Once again it was onwards and upwards! One thing is certain, I could not have done both simultaneously. In the meantime Judith was in an ideal position as a university lecturer to co-ordinate and conduct further research and development into both reflexology and RLD.

As a result of the poster presentation at CAMSTRAND, I was invited to give my first full conference presentation by the National Association of Complementary Therapists in Hospice and Palliative Care (NACTHPC). The speaker before me was a well respected palliative care consultant. His presentation was engaging and empathic, and I was already nervous without the added pressure of having to follow such a polished charismatic speaker! However, I took a deep breath and launched right into it. After all, if I couldn't speak about RLD, who could? As it turns out an audience of therapists and reflexologists is a warm and friendly supportive one.

Members of NACTHPC are therapists and practitioners of different therapy modalities, not just reflexology. One of the members, Janet Le Sueur, a senior MLD practitioner, was asked by the committee for feedback on my presentation. She pointed out that the results were similar to those that might be expected with MLD.

The biggest loss occurs during the first treatment, and results are consolidated during subsequent treatments. This was a very helpful observation and something others have mentioned since. Her written feedback is on the next page.

"As a Lymphoedema Nurse Specialist, I was particularly interested to hear Sally Kay present her research relating her approach to reflexology and lymphoedema.

Sally gave a very engaging and enthusiastic presentation - her sheer joy of the unfolding of the results apparent. Sally presented her findings:

- *How her theory and practice developed*
- *Breast cancer related lymphoedema*
- *Six people who all showed an amazing loss of fluid after their four treatments.*
- *Overview of the MYCaW follow up*
- *Future plans to develop the technique and funding for this development*
- *Sally critically analysed her study and identified some of its limitations. I thought this was such exciting work considering the number of people that are affected with lymphoedema and that working on the feet would be much less invasive for MLD therapy.*

I really hope that the long term results are equally successful. Obviously this is a small study but with such exciting potential. I wish Sally every success and now I want to learn reflexology so that I can access her course.

Good luck Sally"
Janet Le Sueur

Later that year I was honoured to receive my first award, the Federation of Holistic Therapists (FHT) Excellence in Practice Award 2012 for Research and Development, into Reflexology Lymph Drainage (RLD) and the management of secondary lymphoedema in patients affected by treatment for breast cancer.

The FHT is the largest and the leading professional association for therapists in the UK and Ireland. It has thousands of members offering a broad range of specialisms, from sports and remedial therapies to complementary healthcare and holistic beauty treatments.

The following year as an Excellence in Practice award winner, my first article about RLD was published in the *FHT International Therapist*, Issue 104 April 2013.

As people gradually heard about RLD, interest in the new technique grew and in response, the RLD course started to evolve organically. I never saw myself as a natural teacher, but I felt compelled to spread the word and share my passion. Since then RLD training has been well received and put to good use by many reflexologists around the world. On successful completion of a case study, approved RLD reflexologists are listed on the RLD website to help anyone looking for this type of reflexology.

The content of the course is strengthened by the research data, and many case studies from the training underpin the true value of this unique approach.

In recognition for the research and development of RLD, I received further awards from both the International Council of Reflexologists and the Association of Reflexologists (AoR) as well as the prestigious accolade of Honorary Fellowship of the AoR, the UK's largest professional reflexology organisation.

If you believe in something good, keep going and never give up no matter how turbulent the waters. Be led by your dreams. One small step at a time is all it takes to move forward.

Onwards & upwards!

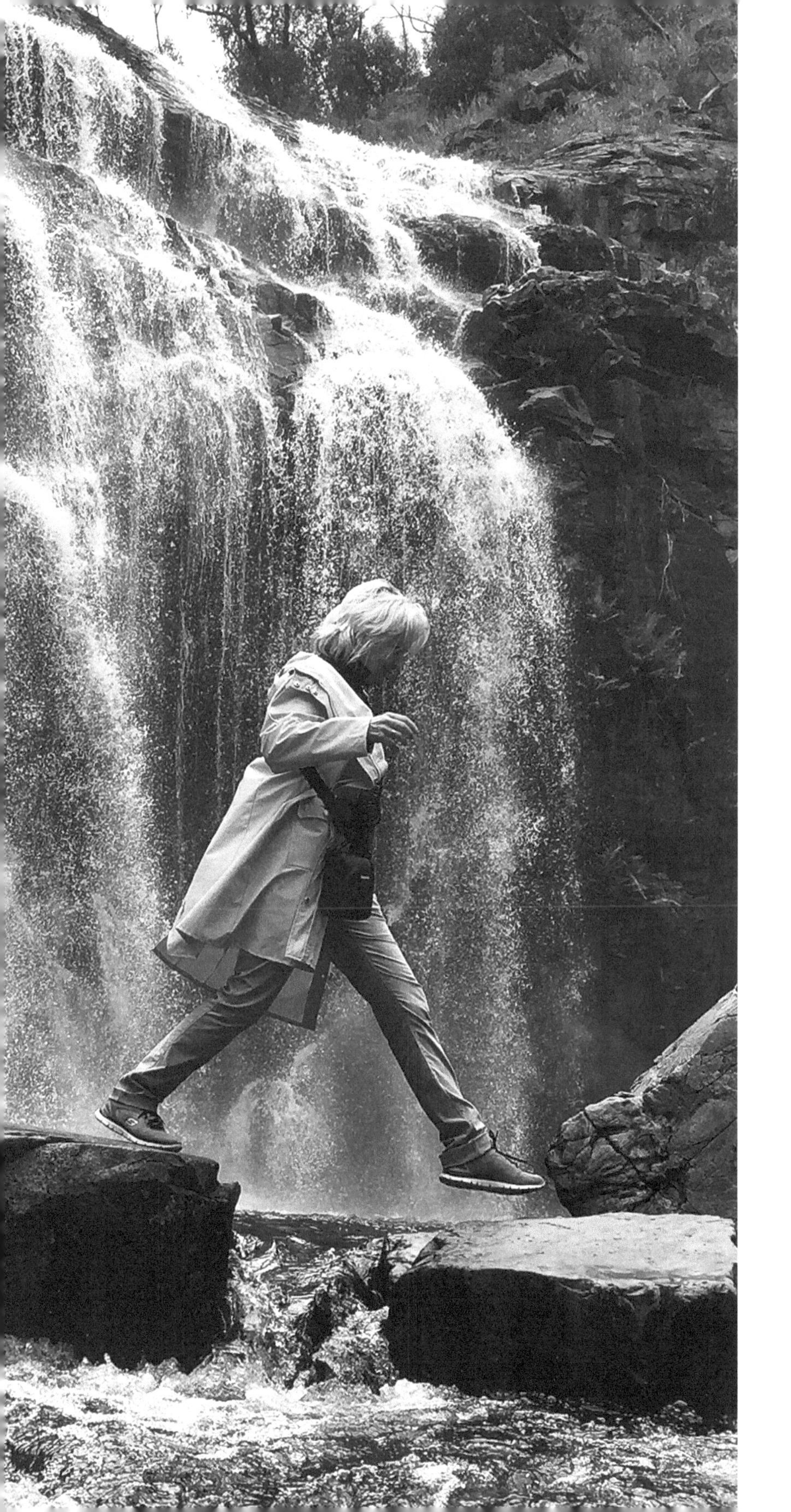

"Every journey
begins with a
single step"
– Lao Tzu

Chapter 2
Small Steps to Research

Expectation

In this chapter I will discuss some of the rationale and challenges of research and data collection. Read about why I believe it's a good idea for all reflexologists to develop an evidence based practice and introduce a simple and effective verified outcome measure. Find out what happened when I did just that!

Why do we need research?

Evidence based reflexology practice is useful for our profession as well as for anyone who is evaluating it.

In general and compared to conventional medicine there is a distinct lack of research evidence in complementary therapies. Yet reflexology has been around for thousands of years and as reflexologists we all know it works. So why do we need scientific proof? What is the value of it to clients and the wider reflexology community? Well in practice there will always be questions about reflexology. For example,

"Does reflexology make a difference?"

"Can reflexology help me with my symptoms?"

In the UK, the current voluntary regulation professional guidelines do not allow reflexologists to claim to treat a condition, because of the lack of evidence. Instead the advice is to treat the client and not the problem. Reflexologists need to be mindful of this in practice and careful not to be misleading with promotional material or website content. Take care not to claim that reflexology can cure a condition when planning a course of treatments and managing expectations of the aims and outcomes.

Then there is the age-old question, "How does reflexology work?"

Unfortunately until we fully understand the mechanism of action of reflexology it's a tough one to answer. The truth is, even though there are multiple theories and beliefs surrounding reflexology, depending on the source, we cannot say for sure how it works. For example, some people believe it unblocks the meridians, or energy pathways, others are sure it is the response of the nervous system, or maybe the circulation or the fascia, while some see it as little more than a placebo.

Does it actually matter? Well, it would be useful to have some research evidence to support any of the theories for reflexology so we could take ownership of the wonderful therapeutic benefits it can bring to the mind, body and spirit.

Another reason for more robust research evidence is the acceptance of reflexology into a wider healthcare setting. Scientific evidence would make it harder to dismiss reflexology as "quackery".

This lack of evidence to prove the benefits means reflexologists are sometimes only able to volunteer their services and be grateful for the experience of this. Indeed volunteering is a very rewarding thing to do. It is a great opportunity to put reflexology to good use and gain valuable experience while helping others. However, this is not sustainable for reflexologists.

Surely this is another reason to look for evidence in support of the therapeutic benefits, so that more reflexologists are paid, valued and respected as integrated healthcare professionals.

Simple data collection

Where do you begin with research?

Most reflexology practitioners are unlikely to be in a position where clinical research is an option, for example working or studying at a university, hospital or in a medical setting. However, if you are involved with a charity, community project or voluntary organisation, data collection can be a helpful tool. By using a verified standard outcome measure to collect information about the services, there is the potential to analyse the data into credible evidence and present the results in testimony of the benefits to service users in support of a funding application.

For reflexologists working as a sole practitioner or as part of a team in a larger organisation, integrating a standard outcome measure into your practice is a good place to start. This is something I highly recommend all reflexologists to try.

A small example of user-friendly standard outcome measures includes the following:

- Visual Analogue Scale (VAS)
- Measure Yourself Medical Outcome Profile (MYMOP)
- Measure Yourself Concerns and Wellbeing (MYCaW)

VAS is the simplest of these. It is a 10cm (100mm) line with a smiley face at one end and sad face at the other. It can be used to assess any presenting condition or more than one concern.

It is usually completed by the client or patient, who puts a mark somewhere on the line depending how they feel about the problem. It is simple to use and there is no pressure because they don't even have to choose a number. To extract the data from a VAS, simply place a ruler on the 10cm line and the score is where the mark lies.

e.g., Pain ☺ ____ ☹

MYMOP, Measure Yourself Medical Outcome Profile, is a patient-generated, individualised, outcome questionnaire. It is problem-specific but includes general wellbeing. It is applicable to everyone who presents with symptoms, whether they are physical, emotional or social. It is brief and simple to administer.

MYCaW, Measure Yourself Concerns and Wellbeing, is an individualised questionnaire that has been designed for evaluating complementary therapies in cancer support care. It may be suitable for use in other settings too.

Both MYMOP & MYCaW use a 0–6 scale to score one or two concerns and wellbeing. MYMOP has some additional questions about problems with "activity", whether physical, social or psychological, and "medication", and whether or not taking it is causing a problem.

For more information about MYMOP and MYCaW, see Useful sources of information on page 227.

All three of these examples, VAS, MYCaW and MYMOP, are easy enough to integrate into a client consultation, and now is a good time to try them! They demonstrate the results to both reflexologist and client and help to evaluate treatment outcomes and furnish an overview of the bigger picture in an audit of services.

Having your own data is advantageous if you are invited to give a talk or small presentation. You can deliver a powerful message when you speak from experience and have some evidence to back it up. Remember, know your audience when giving a talk!

Still not convinced about the merits of data collection, or never want to give a talk, because it's not your thing, you just love working as a hands-on reflexologist? Of course it is fantastic work, and this is a passion shared by the reflexology community. However, there is still a case to answer for collecting data.

When a client feels better, how can we be sure that it was the reflexology and not something else? It is difficult to prove the therapeutic benefits are the effect of the intervention.

The following example of a familiar scenario is a fictitious conversation with a client who has reflexology treatments for back pain.

Reflexologist: "How has your back pain been since your appointment last month?"

Client: "Much better thanks, come to think about it, I haven't taken any painkillers this week, and I've slept better... as you ask, I can't remember when I stopped taking the painkillers."

Was this a coincidence or an effect of the reflexology? Either way it is difficult to prove, and the client may think, "I was getting better anyway".

How much more powerful would the same results be had the client scored their back pain and tiredness (from pain-related lack of sleep) before having reflexology, and the results been directly attributed to the effect of the treatment. By asking the client to score the presenting problem, it can help them to define their main concerns from the beginning. When the pain has eased it's easy to forget just how bad it was. A baseline score is a reminder and a follow-up score can help the client to appreciate the improvements and you to evaluate the outcome of the treatment.

Developing a conceptual framework

Imagine the delight when I realised the RLD results were immediate and measurable. There was a recurring theme in a group of women with a similar problem, who received the same intervention (RLD) and the results provided tangible quantitative data. This was the conceptual framework for the RLD research proposal.

The primary aim of the study was to explore the use of RLD as a physical therapy for the management of breast cancer related lymphoedema. A secondary aim was to explore a correlation between specific lymphatic reflexes of the feet and function of the lymphatic system in the body.

Here's what happened next

Six women who all suffered with breast cancer related lymphoedema in one arm were recruited and agreed to take part in a six-week study.

Appointments were given for them to come along once a week for six weeks at the same time on the same day of the week. Lymphoedema swelling can fluctuate throughout the day. It occurs naturally and is affected by many things, for example, temperature, type of activity or inactivity even. Sticking to the same time of day helps avoid bias of naturally occurring fluctuations.

Week 1

During the first appointment, consent forms and consultation documentation were completed.

Using two different standard outcome measures, Limb Volume Circumference Measurements (LVCM) and MYCaW, to establish the baseline, measurements were taken for both arms, normal and swollen, with the normal arm acting as the control to compare against the swollen arm.

LVCM is done by treating the arm as a cylinder and using a mathematical formula to calculate the volume of a series of 4cm cylinders (see Chapter 8 on page 156).

LVCM only measures the cylinder of the arm, and does not include any swelling in the hand, the shoulder or under the arm or surrounding area of the chest wall or back.

The MYCaW first form was used to record individual concerns and their baseline scores were noted.

Week 2

Both arms were measured before the first RLD treatment and re-measured immediately afterwards.

Week 3

Both arms were measured before the second RLD treatment and re-measured immediately afterwards.

MYCaW concerns were re-scored.

Week 4

Both arms were measured before the third RLD treatment and re-measured immediately afterwards.

Week 5

Both arms were measured before the fourth RLD treatment and re-measured immediately afterwards.

Week 6

Follow-up measurements were taken of both arms and MYCaW forms completed. There was no RLD treatment this week.

All data was scrutinised for accuracy and the results analysed separately for each participant, to explore changes in the arm volume as well as the MYCaW scores.

Week 1: Baseline MYCaW

Participant	Concern 1	Concern 2
P.01	Swelling	Aching
P.02	Swelling	Aching
P.03	Swelling	Aching
P.04	Swelling	Pain
P.05	Cosmetic/wearing a sleeve	Aching
P.06	Swelling	Aching

Table 1: Baseline MYCaW concerns

Once the individual data sets had been collated, organised and understood each case was compared with the others to look for any similarities and recurring themes in the results.

What happened next was quite remarkable: not only did all six of the participants have a statistically significant reduction in swelling but the greatest loss had happened during the first RLD treatment in each case (see Chart 01: Percentage of excess swelling between the swollen arm & the normal arm on page 53 and Chapter 9 on page 167 for more details).

BASELINE					WEEK 1		WEEK 6	
					Difference before	Volume before	Volume loss	Difference after
Participant	Age	Years	R	L	% Arm	ml	ml	%
P.01	62	7	✔		15.4%	358.96	289.34	3%
P.02	53	3	✔		13.9%	366.78	132.07	8.9%
P.03	38	8	✔		19.5%	456.97	269.75	7.9%
P.04	56	4		✔	7.1%	146.03	126.53	0.9%
P.05	48	10		✔	19.5%	425.07	314.49	5.1%
P.06	49	5	✔		9.1%	322.09	270.67	1.5%

Table 2: **Summary**

Baseline summary:

The participant age range was from 38 to 62 years and they had all been living with secondary lymphoedema for between 3 and 10 years. Nobody was newly diagnosed. The right dominant arm was affected in four of the participants and left non-dominant in two cases. In all but one case, P5, the proximal section of the arm was more swollen than the distal.

A few highlights

Participant 1 (P1) was 62 years old and had suffered with lymphoedema for seven years in her right dominant arm which was 15.4% bigger than the normal arm, and contained 358.96ml. By week 6, she had lost 289.34ml of this and her swollen arm was now only 3% bigger and best of all, she felt "normal" again. She had been knitting a shawl for a new grandchild. Before RLD it was a slow process which made her arm ache after knitting only two rows and she would have to stop and rest. With the reduction in swelling she managed to finish the shawl in record time.

Participant 3 (P3) was the youngest in the group at 38 years old, and had suffered with lymphoedema for eight years in her right dominant arm which was 19.5% bigger than the left arm, and contained 456.97ml. That is almost half a litre of fluid. Imagine this as a bottle of water in a handbag, the weight and pressure this puts on the shoulder. She also had a lot of swelling in the deltoid area of the shoulder, above the measurable cylinder of the arm. It was so swollen she had to go up a dress size and even then, clothing fabric had to be stretchy. She was very self-conscious about this. In the third week she arrived for her appointment looking radiant in a new outfit, thrilled to have dropped a dress size because the swelling had reduced so much, and she was positively glowing.

With renewed confidence, and a spring in her step, the next week she joined a gym and started doing Zumba. Previously she had been too self-conscious about the swelling, fearing people would stare at her arm, and this prevented her from exercising. Ironically exercise is good for the management of lymphoedema.

This is a heartwarming example of reflexology giving back control, enabling positive changes and improving quality of life and with this a gift of **hope**.

Participant 4 (P4), who had the least amount of measurable swelling, chose "pain" as a MYCaW concern. This was due to the pocket of lymphoedema swelling under her arm which she referred to as "my tennis ball". Holding her arm away from her body to stop it rubbing caused so much discomfort, that the pain was referred up into the neck and shoulder because she couldn't relax the arm down. During the six weeks her tennis ball disappeared! She only had three RLD sessions, as she missed the third week of the study due to being on holiday. The trip included a four-hour flight each way, and flying can exacerbate lymphoedema swelling, but despite this she managed to maintain the results.

This illustrates why two outcome measures are better than one. It would be easy to assume that less swelling equals less pain, but this is clearly not the case. MYCaW highlights this with additional subjective information about the concerns of the patient.

For Participant 5 (P5) the distal section of her affected swollen arm was much worse than the proximal. She also had a swollen hand and fingers which she described as being like "sausages". She was unable to make a fist. During the first RLD she felt tingling and movement in her fingers and by the end of the session they were more flexible. After four sessions she needed a new compression glove because much of the swelling on the back of her hand had reduced in size and the garment was no longer tight fitting.

Her first MYCaW concern was "cosmetic - wearing the sleeve". She hated the glove part the most because it cannot be hidden with a long sleeve and it gets grubby. Worst of all she minded people asking, "What have you done to your hand?"

From baseline week 1 to before the first RLD treatment in week 2 there is a slight fluctuation in swelling for everyone, which naturally occurs up and down. The increase for Participant 2 (P2) was because she had to drive, something she hadn't done for three years since the mastectomy. Unfortunately her husband was taken ill in the week, and admitted to a hospital an hour's drive away from home. Doing this journey caused more swelling and aching, hence the steep increase.

The results show that everyone experienced the greatest reduction in swelling during the first RLD treatment (in week 2). Subsequent treatments appear to consolidate these results which made a significant difference to all six participants. Consistent results like these have become a familiar pattern.

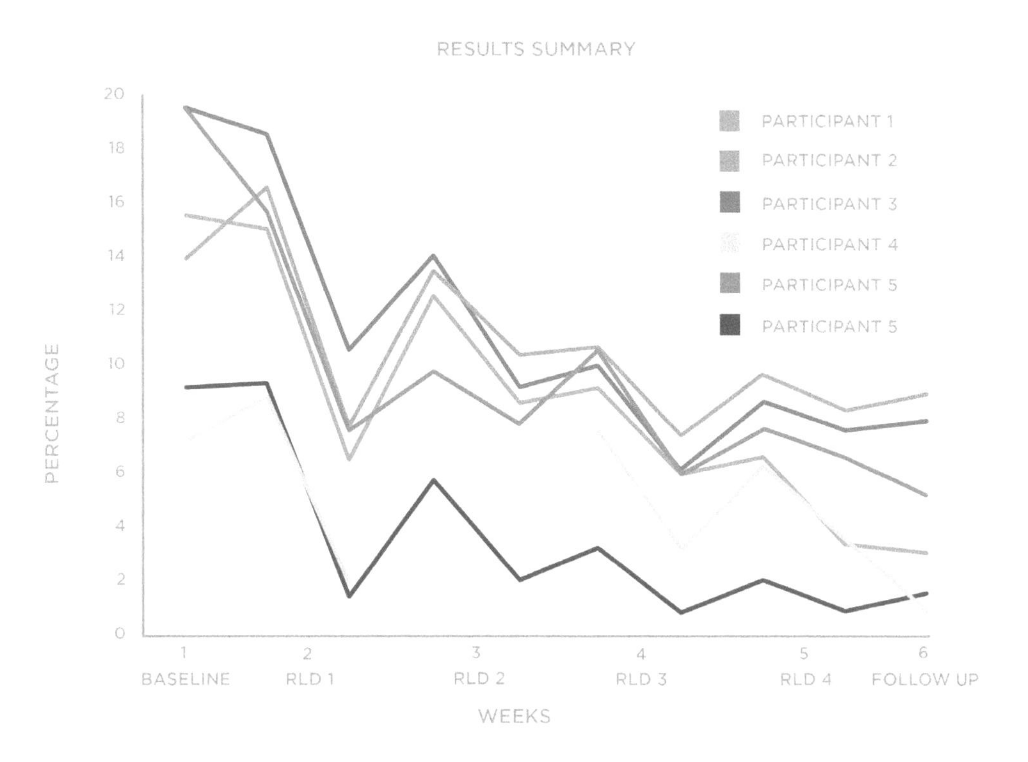

Chart 01: Percentage of excess swelling between the swollen arm & the normal arm

The graph shows the summary of results for each of the participants. For a more detailed insight into the data sets for each individual case see Chapter 9 on page 167.

Statistical analysis of the results of this case series was highly significant and further research was recommended. In 2013 on the strength of these initial findings, Welsh cancer charity Tenovus awarded funding of £12,263.00 for further RLD research, to be conducted in partnership with Cardiff Metropolitan University.

The next step

Twenty-six participants were recruited into the study and the intervention phase was completed between January and June 2014. Two papers have since been published for peer review in *Clinical Practice in Complementary Therapies*, January 2016 and June 2018. See research abstracts in Chapter 9 on page 167.

The overall trend in these results shows similarities to those of the individual participants who took part in the first study. The greatest reduction was during the first RLD treatment and subsequent treatments seem to consolidate these results.

All of the participants had reductions in swelling of the affected arm. All of the statistical tests run on the before and after volumes showed that all effects were statistically significant ($p<.001$).

Subjective scores of participant concerns and wellbeing using MYCaW indicated changes on all three scales to be of clinical significance to the participants. The levels of the primary and secondary concerns were both significantly lower at follow-up when compared to baseline, and participant wellbeing increased significantly from baseline to follow-up. Nobody dropped out during the study and the attrition rate was zero.

In addition to LVCM and MYCaW being used, for data collection a short exit interview was recorded and transcribed. The following are examples of quotes from these.

"...I found the whole thing was one of the top ten highlights of my life"

"...I was really quite sceptical thinking, 'this isn't going to work, but I'll do it anyway', and I was amazed, really totally amazed to see the difference in my hand after the first session. I was just ...I couldn't get over it"

"It's lighter, I haven't got the heaviness, I haven't got the aching in my arm, the swelling has gone down, I can stretch my arm, it just feels a lot better"

"I look at myself in the mirror now and I can see there's an actual shape to my arm whereas before it went straight down"

"I want to continue because I think it's wonderful... I think it's the best thing that's happened"

"It's absolutely amazing because people do suffer with lymphoedema for years and it's so painful, if something as pleasant as this can do something it's wonderful. It's a wonderful, wonderful thing"

In response to the preliminary results of the research reported to Tenovus, the Welsh cancer charity, a further allocation of funding was received to enable follow-up measurements to be taken and get an idea of how long the benefits of RLD are maintained.

Three months after the intervention phase had been completed everyone who participated was invited to a single follow-up appointment where both arms would be re-measured and the volume recalculated. In total 22 of the original 26 participants responded to the invitation to attend one final time. No treatment was given at this appointment.

The intervention phase of the study had taken six months to complete. Re-measuring months later was not part of the original research design and is therefore not included in the research paper.

The disparity of several compounding factors made it difficult to make a case-by-case comparison of the follow-up measurements but the underlying trend was undeniable. Not one participant's affected arm was as swollen as it had been when baseline measurements were taken before receiving the course of four RLD treatments. Everyone had maintained an improvement in the swollen arm.

Depending when participants were involved in the study, the timescale of maintaining the improvement was between three and nine months. Some were delighted to report they hadn't needed to wear the compression sleeve all summer and felt "normal" without it. Others had chosen to seek monthly or six-weekly RLD treatments to maintain their results.

One of the participants had travelled quite a distance to take part in the study. She was so delighted by the improvement to her arm, and so was her breast care consultant when she saw him at a routine appointment. However, she realised none of the local reflexologists were able to offer RLD, and mentioned it to her NHS consultant who funded training in RLD for a local reflexology practitioner. His only stipulation was that she feed back the results to him. Read the participant's testimonial in Chapter 10 on page 186.

There has been a wonderful organic ripple effect from this. The reflexologist receives referrals from the breast care consultant and the participant can maintain the improvements to her arm and surrounding area with regular monthly RLD treatments. After 10 years with lymphoedema she no longer has swelling in her arm or wears a compression sleeve. She describes her arm as "normal".

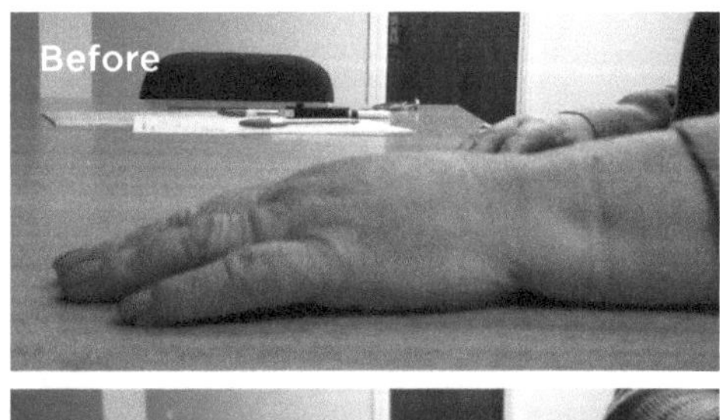

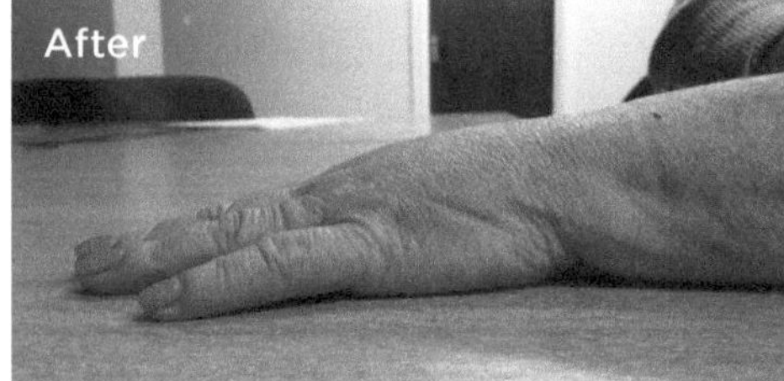

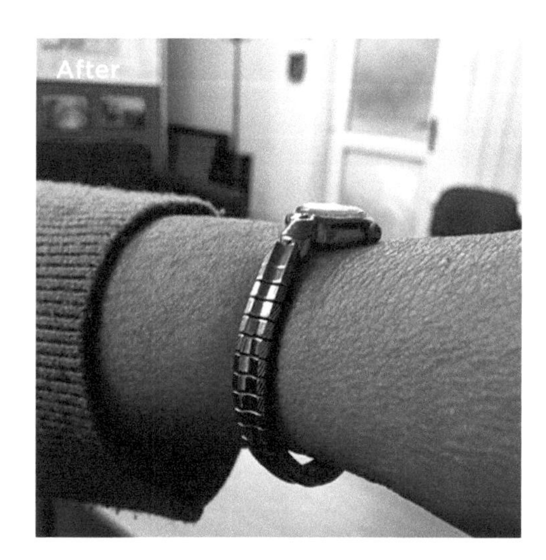

Fig. 06: **Before & After**

The photographs in Fig. 06 were taken immediately before and after one RLD treatment. The mark around the wrist is where the compression sleeve has been worn. This was removed to measure the arm before the RLD. As she took it off she mentioned being unable to wear her rings or watch on this hand at the moment due to the swelling. A reduction in swelling and changes to the skin are clearly visible immediately after RLD. As the arms were re-measured she said, "I wonder if my watch will fit now?" And sure enough it did!

Changes to any swelling in the hand are not included in the arm volume measurements, only the cylinder of the arm is measurable. See How to measure the arm on page 159.

For more details about RLD research, including extracts from the original research proposal and a detailed account of the results as well as published research abstracts, see Chapter 9 on page 167.

Where will the next step lead? Continue your journey with a review of the structure and drainage function of the lymphatic system in the next chapter. It is written for reflexology practitioners to understand why, and how, to reflect this on the reflexes of the feet.

Reflection

- Data collection is good news for clients and practitioners
- Simple user-friendly outcome measures are easy to integrate
- A small case series can form a foundation for future research

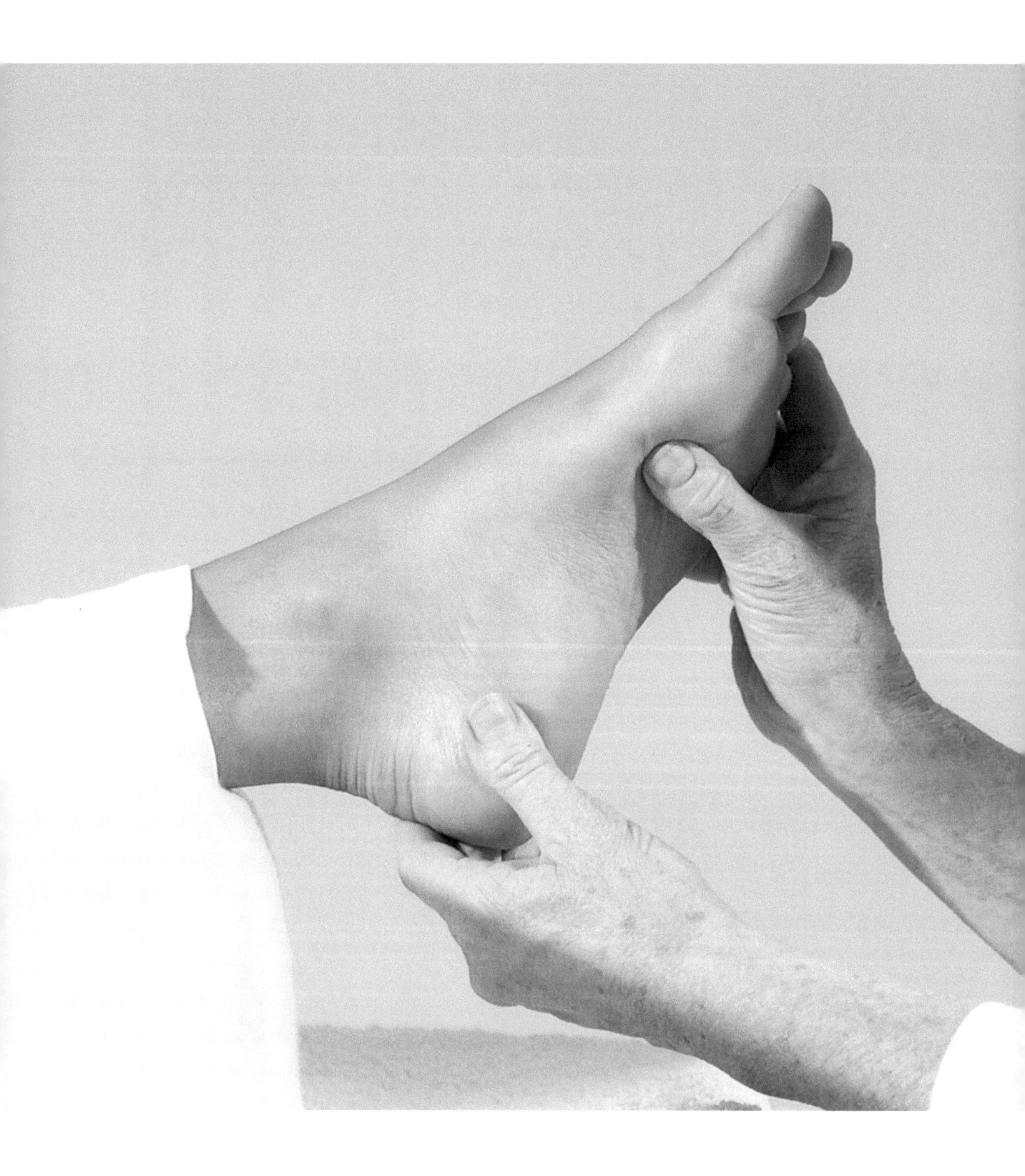

Section 2

FIRST PRINCIPLES OF RLD

Chapter 3
The Lymphatic System

Expectation

This chapter provides an elemental review of the lymphatic system, in both structure and function and its relationship to the first principles of Reflexology Lymph Drainage. This will also help you to understand why the RLD reflexes flow in a prescriptive sequence in order to cause an effect on the drainage function of the body.

The lymphatic system is a one-way drainage system. Its function is transport and defence. It clears proteins, cellular debris, pathogens, fatty acids and other particulate waste matter from the tissues. For the purpose of this chapter the focus is on the drainage rather than the immune function.

In simple terms when the heart pumps arterial oxygenated blood to the cells, plasma is filtered by the blood capillaries and the de-oxygenated blood returned in the veins. Approximately 15-20% of blood plasma will enter the interstitial spaces, instead of the venous return.

Unlike blood circulation, which has a two-way transport system that is pumped by the heart, lymph relies on movement, breathing and gravity to transport it in one direction only. Lymph vessels are compressed by muscular movement, which forces the lymph forward.

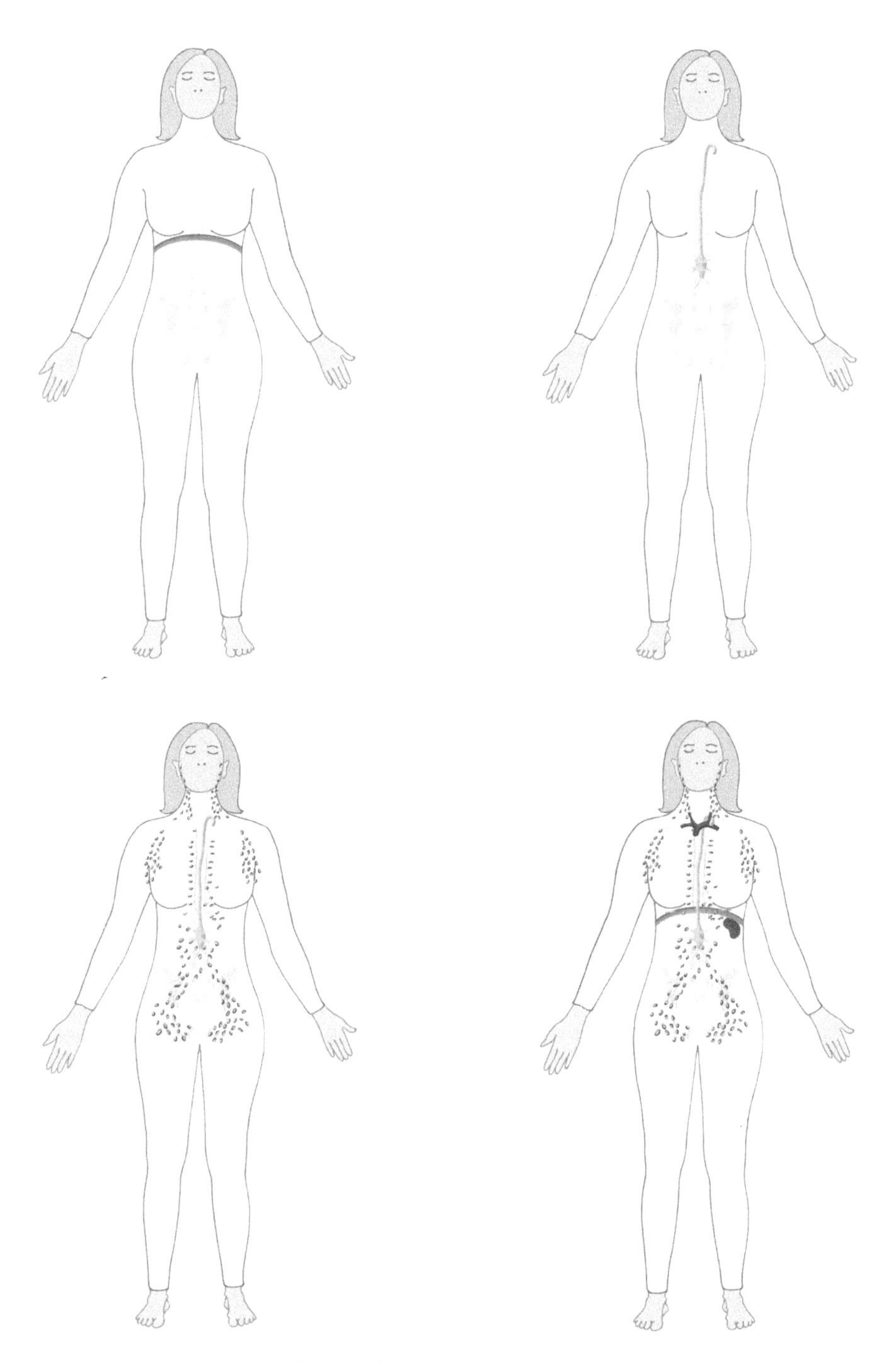

Fig. 07: **The lymphatic system and RLD**

Lymph

Lymph is the fluid from the interstitial spaces which enters the lymphatic system through a network of superficial initial lymphatic capillaries. These are found below the surface of the skin and in the soft tissue of the body.

This is where the lymph's journey begins. It moves away from the cells in lymph vessels towards the lymph nodes where it is filtered before entering larger, deeper lymph vessels. These eventually converge into lymphatic ducts which return the fluid to the blood circulation via the subclavian vein. This is a continuous cycle to maintain a healthy balance of fluid in the body.

Initial lymphatics and lymph vessels

The lymph cell walls of the initial lymph capillaries overlap each other to form a one-way valve. Osmotic pressure allows the waste fluid to enter the lymphatic system and the overlapping cells prevent it from flowing back out via the capillary walls.

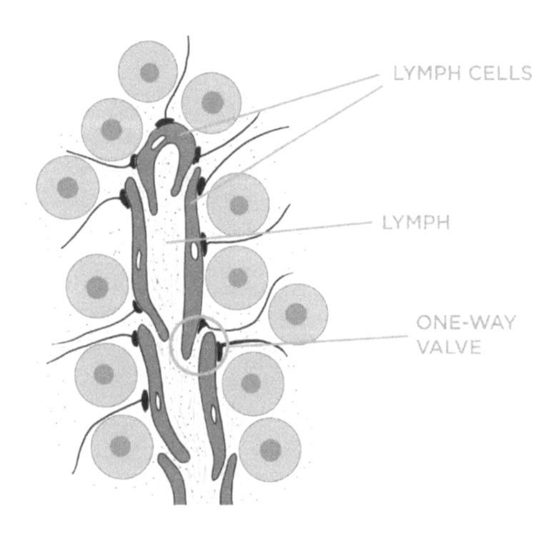

Fig. 08: **Initial lymph capillary**

The initial lymphatics merge with lymph vessels that gradually increase in size and they have slightly thicker walls. Lymph is carried away from the cells towards the lymph nodes. The larger lymph vessels have a series of bicuspid valves to prevent backflow and keep the lymph moving in one direction towards the blood circulation. Afferent lymph vessels enter the surface of the node in several places where valves open inwards. See Fig. 09: Lymph node on page 63.

Lymph nodes and larger lymph vessels

All lymph is filtered through at least one lymph node before it can return back into the circulatory system via the subclavian vein.

There are believed to be between 600 and 700 lymph nodes in the human body, with approximately 160 of them situated in the neck (cervical lymph nodes). Nodes are oval structures and they may vary in size. They are densely packed with white blood cells, including macrophages and lymphocytes.

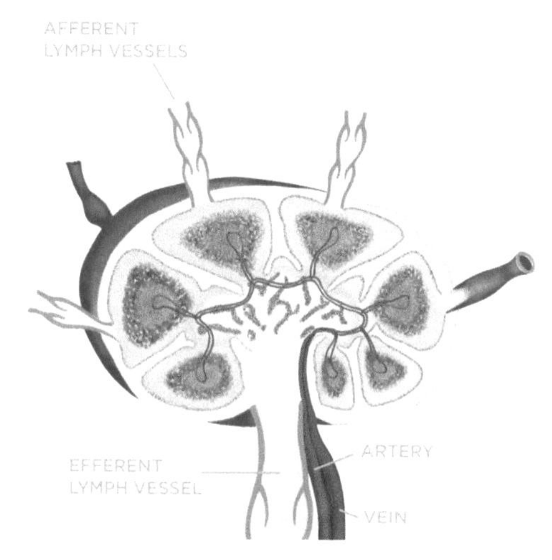

Fig. 09: Lymph node

As the lymph passes through the node it is filtered for pathogens, antigens and other cellular debris and this is destroyed by phagocytosis.

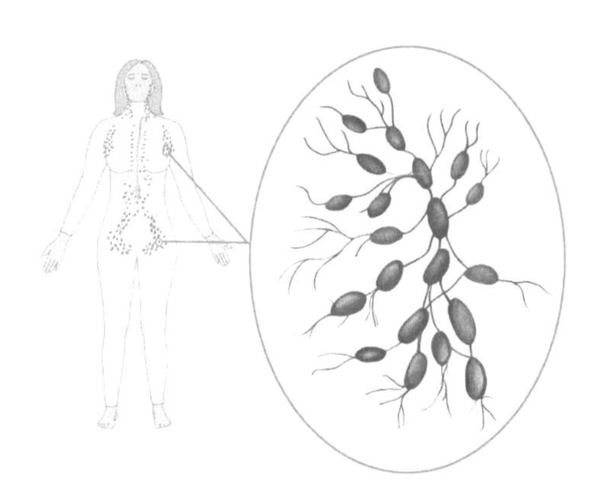

Fig. 10: Lymph nodes

Once the lymph has been filtered, larger efferent lymph vessels transport the lymph out of the node, either towards other nodes or into larger, deeper vessels. Eventually the lymph vessels merge into large lymphatic pathways and these converge at the subclavian vein where fluid is returned back into the blood circulation (see Fig. 12: Subclavian vein on page on page 233).

Thoracic duct and cisterna chyli

The thoracic duct is the largest lymphatic vessel. It ascends vertically along the thoracic vertebrae in the chest and curves in towards the left subclavian vein, returning lymph fluid to the blood circulation. Lymph is transported upwards from the lower part of the body via the thoracic duct.

Anatomically the thoracic duct ascends the length of the 12 thoracic vertebrae from T-12 to T-1. Adjoining this below is the cisterna chyli situated in line with the first and second lumbar vertebrae, L-1 and L-2.

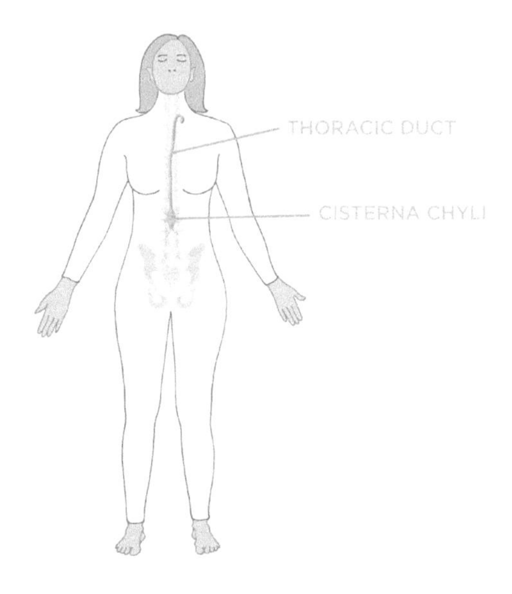

Fig. 11: **Cisterna chyli & thoracic duct**

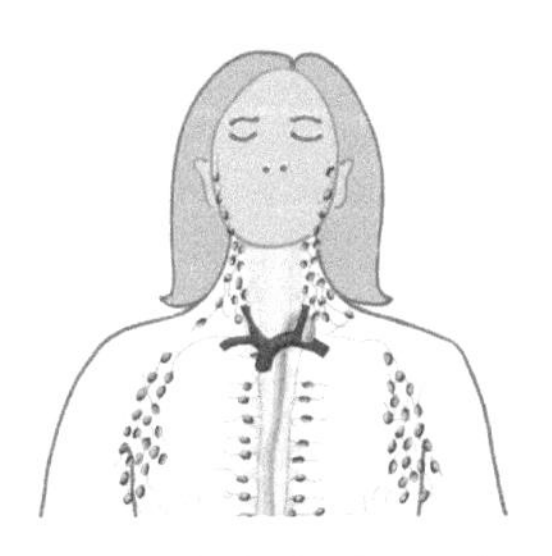

Fig. 12: **Subclavian vein**

The cisterna chyli collects lymph from the intestine, abdominal organs and legs. It acts as a small reservoir which collects and stores the lymph before it travels up the thoracic duct to the left lymphatic duct and which empties into the left subclavian vein.

Using the anatomical reflection theory, the cisterna chyli reflex sits in the medial edge of the cuneiform bone and the thoracic duct runs the length of the medial edge of the first metatarsal.

Right and left drainage

The lymphatic system does not drain equally on the left and right side of the body.

The right side drains lymph from the right side of the head and neck, the right arm and the right upper quadrant of the body. This lymph is returned to the blood circulation via the right lymphatic duct which empties into the right subclavian vein.

The left side drains lymph from the left side of the head and neck, the left arm, the left upper quadrant, the abdomen and the left and right leg. Lymph returns to the blood circulation via the left lymphatic duct which empties into the left subclavian vein.

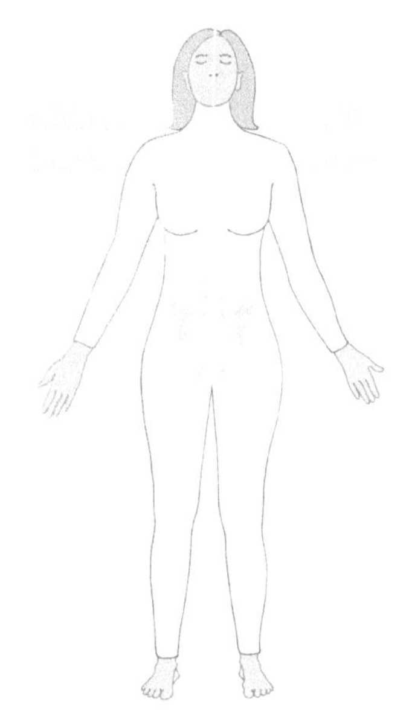

Fig. 13: Right & left drainage

Spleen

The spleen is the largest organ of the lymphatic system. The spleen filters the blood for old or damaged red blood cells, platelets and pathogens and antigens. Phagocytosis metabolises these in the spleen.

The spleen reflex is included at the end in the RLD sequence with the intention to boost the phagocytosis function in the removal of stagnant cellular debris.

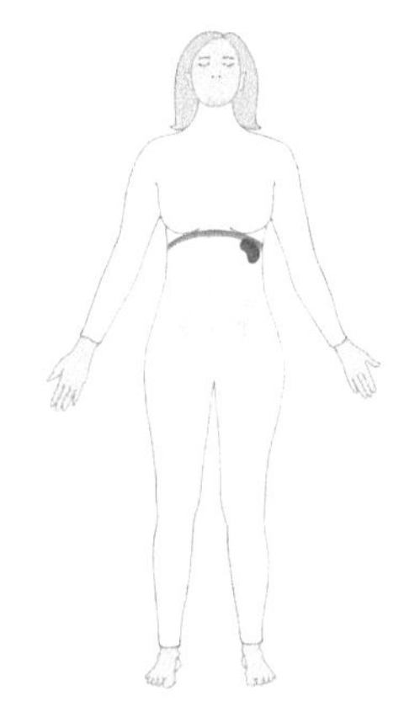

Fig. 14: Spleen

Other organs of the system

The other parts of the lymphatic system include tonsils, the thymus, Peyer's patches and bone marrow but the function of these parts relates to the immune response rather than a drainage action and as such they are not included in the RLD sequence. However, their function may well be affected by the treatment.

The function of the thymus gland is most active from infancy through childhood and puberty to adult maturity after which it begins to shrink. The immune function of the thymus is to produce T lymphocytes. These T cells are antibodies that help to recognise and destroy pathogens and antigens.

The function of the tonsils is to produce lymphocytes and antibodies and strategically protect against the invasion of pathogens and antigens. They are large lymphatic nodules embedded in mucous membrane, found in the oral cavity and the pharynx.

Bone marrow produces lymphocytes and is considered to be a component of the lymphatic system.

Peyer's patches are found in the wall of the ileum and contain macrophages that capture and destroy bacteria to prevent a breach of the intestinal wall.

Lymph flow

Movement of lymph in the lymphatic system is continuous. Lymph flows along the pathways in one direction and does not normally take a diversion or find a new route. To cause an effect on the drainage action of the system, a space must be created in order to draw the fluid from one area of the body to another, like a vacuum.

As a visual learner, I liken this process to the plumbing in the house. If you want to draw more water in from the mains outside the house, first you need to turn the tap on for water to exit the system into the drain. It is not possible for more water to come into the house until this space has been created. I see the lymphatic system similarly. Therefore, it is important to get everything moving towards the subclavian vein (the tap and the drain) so that space is created in the system for more fluid to be drawn into the initial lymphatic vessels from the interstitial spaces.

We all know what happens when plumbing goes wrong! And it's the same for the human body. We will explore this further in the next chapter.

Reflection

- The structure of the lymphatic system provides the means for lymph drainage to flow in one direction
- The function of the system helps to maintain a healthy balance of fluid in the body
- The left and right side of the body do not drain equally
- Space must be created to cause an effect on the drainage function

Chapter 4
Lymphoedema

Expectation

In this chapter find out what happens when the drainage function of the lymphatic system is interrupted and discover why lymphoedema swelling can develop.

What is lymphoedema?

Lymphoedema is a chronic condition which causes tissue swelling when interstitial fluid accumulates because of blocked, damaged or absent lymph drainage channels.

Lymphoedema is a progressive and debilitating condition for which no cure is currently available. It can be painful and incapacitating, as well as restricting the mobility and range of movement in the affected area. There are two classifications of lymphoedema, primary and secondary.

Primary lymphoedema

Primary lymphoedema is caused by an intrinsic hereditary congenital defect of the lymphatic system. This can affect the lymph vessels or the lymph nodes or both. Primary lymphoedema may present and develop at birth or during infancy but more commonly it is likely to occur later in life at times of hormonal changes, such as puberty, pregnancy or the menopause.

Developing primary lymphoedema generally follows a familial pattern. It is most likely to start at the same stage of life as it did for the mother or grandmother. For example, if the symptoms began with the onset of the menopause, they are more likely to begin similarly in the next generation. See the testimonial by Dorothy in Chapter 10 on page 186.

Secondary lymphoedema

Secondary lymphoedema is caused by an extrinsic factor, damage to the lymphatic system. This could be caused by surgery, radiation, scar tissue, trauma from accidents, injury and insect bites.

Cancer causes of secondary lymphoedema include surgery and the removal of lymph nodes, damage to lymph vessels, scarring and radiotherapy tissue damage. The site of the tumour and progression of the disease can also cause lymphoedema swelling.

Damage to the lymphatic pathways prevents the lymph from being removed and this causes an excessive build-up of protein-rich interstitial fluid, which is lymphoedema swelling. Once lymph nodes have been removed there is a lifetime risk of developing it.

When lymph nodes are removed the flow of drainage is interrupted, and the lymph begins to build up into lymphoedema. The lack of drainage and subsequent build-up of proteins for a prolonged period of time can lead to the development of fibrosis, the hardening of the tissue fibres. When this happens the affected area feels hard and the swelling is not soft to the touch any more. It becomes more difficult to manage the condition and there is an increased risk of infection.

Symptoms of lymphoedema

Swelling is the main symptom of lymphoedema, in all or part of a limb or in another part of the body. Clothing and jewellery feels tight and this can be difficult to adjust to. Initially the swelling may fluctuate, for example it can get worse during the day and go down again overnight. Lymphoedema swelling usually builds up gradually and becomes more persistent and severe over a prolonged period of time.

The psychological side effects of the symptoms can be devastating on self-confidence and quality of life, as seen in the small sample of participants in Chapter 2 on page 42 and Chapter 9 on page 167. Each person was affected in different yet similar ways. These were both physical and psychological, and one influences the other. When everyday living activities are hampered by the swelling, due to pain or weakness, there is a knock-on effect on quality of life. All this is on top of everything else they have been through since the cancer diagnosis, treatment, recovery, fear and worry about survivorship. Lymphoedema and everything that goes with it is a constant reminder and, in some cases, feels like the final straw.

I have heard plenty of people say, "It's the first thing I think about when I wake up and the last thing before I go to sleep." The heaviness and aching are often likened to constant nagging toothache with no chance of finding relief. "It's taking over my life!"

Physiological and psychological side effects can include:

- Pain, heaviness and aching
- Distorted limb shape
- Impaired function, weakness and reduced mobility or range of movement
- Decreased elasticity and mobility of skin
- Fibrosis
- Dry skin
- Acute inflammatory episodes, recurring bouts of cellulitis
- Anxiety and depression
- Loss of confidence
- Altered body image
- Uncomfortable wearing certain clothing
- Altered ability to complete everyday tasks, employment and leisure activities

Breast cancer related lymphoedema (BCRL - secondary lymphoedema)

Breast cancer is the most common form of cancer in the UK. According to Cancer Research UK (2011), the lifetime risk of developing it is 1 in 8 for women and 1 in 1014 for men in the UK. Approximately 20% of patients develop secondary lymphoedema of the arm following treatment for breast cancer that includes surgery or radiotherapy to the axillary lymph nodes. Once lymph nodes have been removed there is a lifetime risk of developing it. Some people are affected by lymphoedema immediately after treatment, while others may not develop it for months or years and some will never be affected.

Treatment for breast cancer can vary greatly, depending on the stage and progression of the disease. It can range from a lumpectomy, without the removal of any lymph nodes, to a mastectomy and a full clearance of the axillary lymph nodes followed by chemotherapy and/or radiotherapy.

A frequently asked question is, "Can RLD be given to patients who are undergoing a course of chemotherapy treatment?" Unfortunately the answer is not straightforward because there are too many variables and everyone is different.

Cycles of different types of chemotherapy vary, from tablet form to intravenous infusion and from person to person, depending on the dosage and type and how they cope with it. Make an informed choice about how best to adapt any form of reflexology in these circumstances.

When working with patients undergoing chemotherapy treatment, I would not recommend RLD immediately afterwards, as these cytotoxic drugs have a job to do! Providing the client feels well enough, the optimum time for RLD in the chemotherapy cycle is a day or two before. In addition to those who took part in the research, other people often say they feel quite energised after an RLD treatment. I believe that feeling relaxed and energised would be a good starting point for a cycle of chemotherapy.

When planning any reflexology treatment for patients and clients, remember no two people are the same. It is important to consider the individual and all aspects of their wellbeing and current state of health, the stage of the disease, how they are coping with the treatment, recovery from surgery as well as other influencing factors. Sometimes a shorter, gentle relaxing sequence can be enough to bring comfort and support and take the edge off the anxiety at a challenging time.

A useful resource for further information about working as a complementary therapist with people who have been diagnosed with cancer is a book by Dr Peter Mackereth & Ann Carter, *Massage & Bodywork: Adapting Therapies for Cancer Care*. They have a collective wealth of experience and knowledge, which is shared in this very useful book that I often referred to in my early days of working in cancer care.

For up-to-date information about the different stages of treatment as well as the different treatments for breast cancer, use a reliable website, such as NHS, Cancer Research UK, or Macmillan.

When lymphoedema swelling develops in the arm, more lymphoedema swelling is often present in the adjacent areas of the body. It is quite common to have a pocket of fluid under the arm which bulges out and causes discomfort along with swelling in the breast area and upper back. This was evident in the research participant who described underarm swelling as "my tennis ball". In one of the testimonials someone else describes it as a "suitcase" which shrank to a "clutch bag" (see Chapter 10 on page 186).

This is something I have frequently seen in patients who receive RLD, and often, afterwards they say, "it feels normal again", and the underarm swelling can disappear in just one treatment. In some cases this swelling is present in people who don't even consider themselves to have lymphoedema because they have no measurable swelling in the arm.

Many of those who are affected by lymphoedema in the arm will also have swelling in the shoulder area, the breast, site of the scar and around the back. This makes clothing uncomfortable to wear. Some people are afraid that wearing the compression garment may exacerbate swelling in the surrounding area. Even so it is important to follow the recommendations of the lymphoedema service.

These photographs were taken before and after one RLD treatment. The lateral aspect clearly shows a pulling around the back of the underarm area before, and afterwards the crease has gone (See Fig. 15).

The posterior view also indicates a reduction in swelling (See Fig. 16).

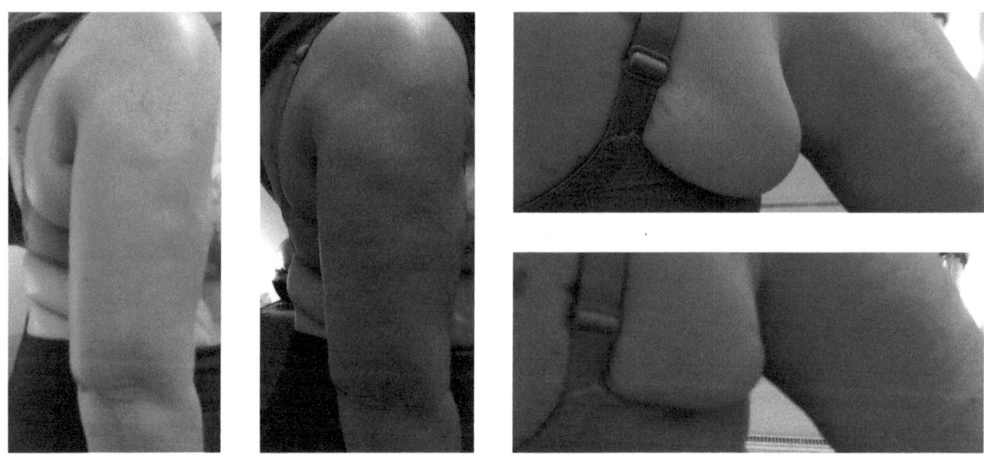

Fig. 15: **Lateral view (Before & After)**

Fig. 16: **Posterior view (Before & After)**

Now that you have learnt about lymphoedema the next chapter explains how the condition is currently managed.

Reflection

- Classifications of lymphoedema are primary and secondary
- Lymphoedema can happen when the drainage channels are blocked or missing
- The symptoms and side effects of lymphoedema swelling cause physical and psychological problems which impact on quality of life

Lymphoedema poem

Lymphoedema can have a devastating effect on breast cancer survivors, physically and emotionally. This touching poem was written by one of the participants in the research. After being diagnosed with cancer she joined cancer charity Tenovus' "Write With Us" group which is one of their support services. She went on to write and successfully publish several children's books.

Lymphoedema

I knew it could happen, but then I forgot
Until someone pointed it out
My arm was quite swollen, my fingers as well
Lymphoedema there could be no doubt

Just a year and a half down the line it had been
So I should have been much more prepared
The clinic provided both mitten and sleeve
And my worries were openly aired

The lymphatic system now needs to be drained
And some things I had to be shown
Exercise, massage and special skin care
But now I do daily alone

In spite of reluctant acceptance of this
As these garments have to compress
In helping the lymph's circulatory flow
Now, part of my life, I confess

With a few broken nails and quite a bruised chin
Through stretching the sleeve up my arm
Now fully aware of new hazards ahead
Could actually do me more harm

Not wearing my rings did upset me the most
But I have an alternative hand
So when in glad rags, my mittens removed
Revealing my gold wedding band

S. Davies

Chapter 5
Management of Lymphoedema

Expectation

This chapter is a summary of the treatments that are currently recommended for people who have been diagnosed with lymphoedema. With no cure available, the options are limited to managing the symptoms which were described in the previous chapter. One of the treatments is Manual Lymph Drainage, a specialist form of massage. Reflexology Lymph Drainage is based on MLD principles.

As previously mentioned in this book, once lymph nodes have been removed there is a lifetime risk of developing lymphoedema. There are guidelines for prevention and self-care, which are recommended for anyone at risk of developing it, or to help prevent the swelling getting worse.

Together with a self-care daily routine, treatment of lymphoedema is known as Decongestive Lymphatic Therapy (DLT). The aim of this is to help to control the symptoms and manage the swelling. There are four main components of DLT and these include skin care, exercise, compression and Manual Lymph Drainage.

When the rudiments of MLD and SLD are understood, they are mirrored onto the reflexes of the feet to reflect the first principles of RLD. You can read more about this in the next chapter.

Prevention and self-care

Simple steps are recommended for anyone who is at risk of developing lymphoedema, or to help to prevent the swelling from getting worse.

- Avoid carrying heavy loads, including a heavy handbag!
- Avoid blood pressure cuffs and injections in the affected limb
- Avoid sunburn and use a high factor sunscreen
- Avoid saunas and hot water on the skin
- Use an insect repellent to avoid insect bites
- Protect the hand and arm, wearing rubber gloves for jobs in the house and heavy duty gardening gloves when gardening
- Drink plenty of water and keep hydrated
- Eat a balanced diet and avoid excess weight
- Take regular "comfortable" exercise

For more information see Lymphoedema Support Network (LSN) in the Useful sources of information on page 227.

Skin care

The swelling causes the skin to stretch and become more susceptible to infections, bacterial, viral or fungal. The texture of skin can change: it might feel thicker, dry and cracked. This can increase the risk of infection and cellulitis. Damaged lymphatic pathways and absence of lymph nodes make it difficult for the immune function to protect against or to help fight infection present in the affected limb. Cellulitis can cause lymphoedema, as well as make the swelling worse.

Special skin care as a preventative measure can help to avoid cellulitis and involves a few basic steps, good personal hygiene and regularly moisturising the skin. Take care to avoid cuts, abrasions, burns or insect bites and in the event of skin damage clean up with antiseptic. Seek medical help for any signs of infection.

Cellulitis, also known as an acute inflammatory episode, is a bacterial infection causing inflamed skin or a rash, heat, swelling and pain, and severe symptoms are flu-like. It is treated with antibiotics. Sometimes visible symptoms disappear but the person still feels unwell. In other cases people are more susceptible to repeated episodes, and for this, a low dose of antibiotics is prescribed as a preventative measure.

RLD treatment is contra-indicated in cases when people are suffering an episode of cellulitis, as is wearing compression garments, MLD, and SLD exercises. Once the cellulitis has cleared up then RLD treatments may resume.

Understanding the pathology of a disease, symptom or side effect will help a reflexology practitioner assess client suitability for a safe reflexology treatment. In cases of cellulitis RLD is contra-indicated because of the risk of spreading any localised infection.

Exercise

Movement of the muscles helps to move and drain the lymph in the body. Recreational gentle exercise, such as walking, yoga, Pilates, swimming or cycling will all help.

One of the big problems with lymphoedema swelling is loss of confidence, and consequently a lack of motivation to exercise. An example of this can be found in Chapter 2 on page 42 and in the case studies in Chapter 10 on page 186. When the swelling was reduced the youngest participant joined a gym and started doing a Zumba class as well as going swimming. As the swelling went down her confidence grew. The wonderful ripple effect of RLD and it's a win-win!

The repetitive action of some daily living activities can cause the swollen limb to ache, things like ironing, vacuuming, cleaning windows, cleaning the bathroom or dusting. This also featured in the research with ironing (see Chapter 2 on page 42 and Chapter 9 on page 167). When the swelling reduced, it was possible to do all the ironing in one go without having to stop and rest between garments with the ironing board up all day!

It is often the small things that make the biggest difference to quality of life, when something makes you feel "normal" again.

Compression garments and bandaging

Compression garments are used to support and protect the skin, promote the muscle pump effect and prevent the accumulation of fluid. They are made from elasticated fabric, and are usually worn as a full sleeve, half sleeve, glove or combination, such as sleeve and glove. Patients who are diagnosed with lymphoedema will be referred to their local lymphoedema clinic and measured and fitted for a compression garment.

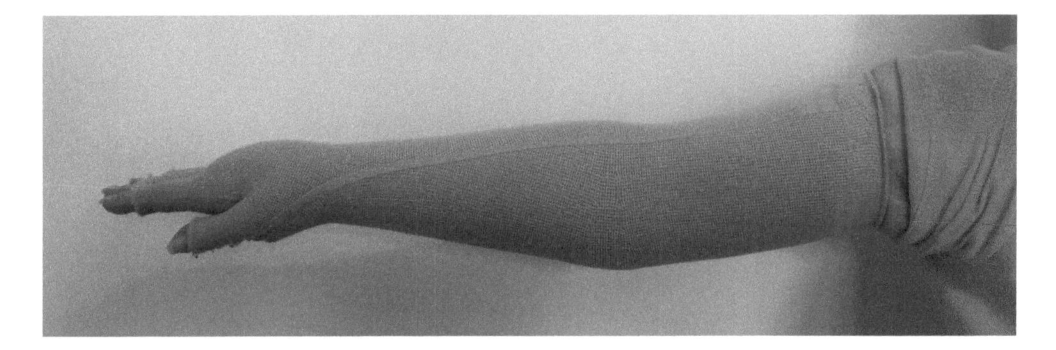

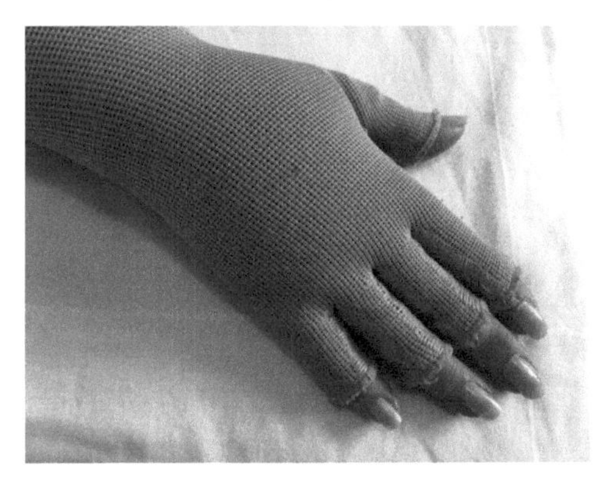

Fig. 17: **Compression garment**

Garments need to feel comfortable, to be firm and provide enough pressure without being too tight.

I have worked with many people with lymphoedema, during the research and in practice, and the general consensus is that people do not like wearing their compression garments, as the following quotes suggest.

"It's like a constant reminder of the breast cancer"

"It's hot and itchy in the summer and shows if I wear short sleeves"

"It's like having a label that says I've only got one breast"

"I hate it when people ask what I've done to my arm"

Some people are compliant and routinely wear their compression garments, despite them being difficult to put on, as was so poignantly described in the poem in the last chapter. They can be unsightly and attract unwanted attention, and people feel uncomfortable and very self-conscious.

Another problem for many people is "what to wear". When clothing gets too tight in the arm because of the swelling, it's no longer suitable because it doesn't fit. People say they end up buying a bigger size just to accommodate the swollen arm and the clothes are too big everywhere else or the choice of clothing is limited to stretchy fabric. After all that messing about and limited choice, nothing feels nice! (See Case study 9: Breast cancer related lymphoedema case study by Sally Kay on page 207.)

Many people affected by secondary lymphoedema do not like wearing the compression garments for a variety of personal reasons. Some are compliant but others prefer not to wear them because of the stigma and discomfort. Initially people are more likely to be compliant, but in time they get fed up with it, leaving it off for a day or two, and don't go back to wearing it.

All of this has a corrosive effect on quality of life!

Multi-layer lymphoedema bandaging

Multi-layer lymphoedema bandaging (MLLB) is for severe cases and is unlikely to be seen in reflexology practice, but it's useful to be informed if a client should mention it.

The aim of bandaging is to help to drain the excess lymph away from the affected area, reduce the swelling and improve the shape. This is only available from specially trained lymphoedema therapists. This type of treatment is extremely labour intensive and time consuming. Unfortunately, it is not readily available in all parts of the UK.

Information is available from the Lymphoedema Support Network and the British Lymphology Society about the centres that are able to provide this type of specialist intensive treatment for lymphoedema.

If intensive multi-layer bandaging treatment is needed, MLD massage may be given before, and then the bandages are applied to prevent the area from refilling.

Manual Lymph Drainage

Manual Lymph Drainage (MLD) is a very gentle form of specialist massage that uses a light pressure. It is not a deep massage because deeper work can flatten the smaller superficial lymph vessels and prevent the fluid from draining away from the tissues. Therefore, RLD is a gentle treatment using light pressure to stimulate the corresponding reflexes.

Natural drainage and flow of the lymphatic system travels in one direction and is unlikely to re-route itself elsewhere in the body. Imagine a blocked stream where the water builds up and pools. With some encouragement it finds a new route, and a new pathway is established.

The aim of MLD for lymphoedema is to reduce the swelling by diverting fluid away from the blockage (the site of missing lymph nodes and/or damaged pathways), to the nearest area on the body where the lymph nodes are fully functional. To do this, space is created with MLD massage in the area of the body that lymph is to be diverted towards. This differs from case to case because the starting point depends on where the swelling or blockage is.

MLD massage for unilateral secondary lymphoedema of the arm begins on the non-swollen, unaffected side of the body to create an empty space and make room for the excess lymph.

For example, if the swelling is in the left arm, the first MLD moves clear the lymphatics on the right side to create space. Next, these moves are repeated on the swollen left side to divert the fluid towards the empty right side where the nodes are working. To finish the massage, MLD moves are repeated on the non-swollen right side again. This helps the stagnant lymph to drain away and increases the flow of lymph in the circulation.

MLD for swelling in the **left arm** is right - left - right

MLD for swelling in the **right arm** is left - right - left

The severity of the swelling determines the extent of treatment required to manage the condition. Not everyone will need MLD, and mild cases can be managed with skin care, exercise and a compression garment.

For severe cases, MLD may be performed daily, or a few times a week for up to six weeks. This is combined with multi-layer bandaging. Afterwards compression garments are worn to prevent further build-up.

Early development of MLD massage techniques was by Dr Vodder in the 1930s. The aim was to improve the function of the lymphatic system. These original techniques were not developed to help reduce lymphoedema, the aim was to purify the body.

Today, some of the different methods of MLD training available include Vodder, Leduc, Földi and Casley-Smith. MLD practitioners will have a recognised qualification in one of these methods. Unfortunately MLD is not always available on the National Health Service. See the Lymphoedema Support Network and the British Lymphology Society for a list of skilled therapists in your area.

Simple Lymph Drainage

Simple Lymph Drainage (SLD) is a very simple self-help, lymph drainage massage type of exercise that can be done by the individual. In principle it is a simple basic version of MLD. It is performed on the skin using a light pressure with the flat fingers or the flat of the hand. The technique is very gentle and should not cause any redness or discomfort to the skin.

There is more than one method of performing SLD, and like MLD all are slight variations of the same theme.

Simple Lymph Drainage typically uses the following principles:

1. Take 5 deep (comfy) breaths as described on page 86 (this gets things moving) - The deep diaphragmatic breathing works the diaphragm muscle. Changes in pressure, caused by deep breathing, encourage the flow of lymph in the deeper lymph vessels. The movement of the deeper vessels in turn allows the initial lymphatics to collect more fluid from the interstitial spaces.

RLD starts by working the diaphragm reflex 5 x

2. Gently stretching the skin at the neck - This is to stimulate the lymph nodes in the neck and encourage movement as they empty and drain away.

RLD works the cervical lymph nodes reflexes

3. Gentle pressure above the collar bone - This is to encourage the right and left lymphatic ducts to empty into the subclavian vein, which in turn creates movement in the deeper lymphatic vessels and space for more fluid to enter the initial lymphatics.

RLD works the subclavian reflex early in the sequence and repeatedly throughout

4. Gentle pressure to the upper lymphatics on the non-swollen side - Clearing a space on the good side to make room for the lymph from the damaged side to filter and drain in the direction of the nearest functioning area of lymph nodes.

5. Clear the non-swollen side - Gently and methodically working across the chest, under the arm and shoulder area.

Once the non-swollen side has been cleared, move on to the swollen side and repeat the moves before returning to the non-swollen side to repeat the moves for a third time. This is the reason RLD begins with the foot on the good side.

SLD self-help DVDs are available from the Lymphoedema Support Network www.lymphoedema.org

Before we move on, let's pause for a breath and think about what it means to "take five deep breaths". Something we take for granted but this can be a challenging frightening instruction for anyone with breathing difficulties or anxiety. For more information about integrating breathing techniques in reflexology see Mackereth, Maycock & Tomlinson, 2017 (full details can be found in Useful sources of information on page 227).

Here Peter Mackereth explains how to enable a comfy breath during reflexology.

"I usually engage with breathing via lung presses or solar plexus areas - I really like suggesting that the person push their feet gently against my forearms or thumbs as they take a comfy rather than deep breath - this can be scary for people with any kind of breathing difficulties - the patient pushes so that they are in control (also this engages their abdominal, leg and calf muscles which encourages further drainage). I usually offer a little resistance and encouragement to gently push as they breathe in and and then 'soften and sink back into the pillows' as they take a slower comfy exhale. On the 5th breath I suggest a 'sniff' at the top of the inhale and then immediately after exhale a little 'huff' (as if misting up a mirror with a pushed exhale) to maximise the exhale comfortably. I usually add in 'if you need to breathe in and out in between the guided breaths, no worries I will work around your pace of breathing'. I say I will breathe also do the 5 Comfy Breaths, and do the sniff and huff along with the technique so they can hear the process so that it is a shared activity."

Essentially the principles of MLD and SLD are the foundation of RLD when it is applied to the reflexes of the feet (and hands). Find out more about this and how each reflex is worked in sequence in the next chapter.

Reflection

- No cure is available for lymphoedema
- Simple steps can be taken to prevent lymphoedema from developing or getting worse
- Management of lymphoedema consists of skin care, exercise, compression and Manual Lymph Drainage
- Reducing the swelling can greatly improve quality of life

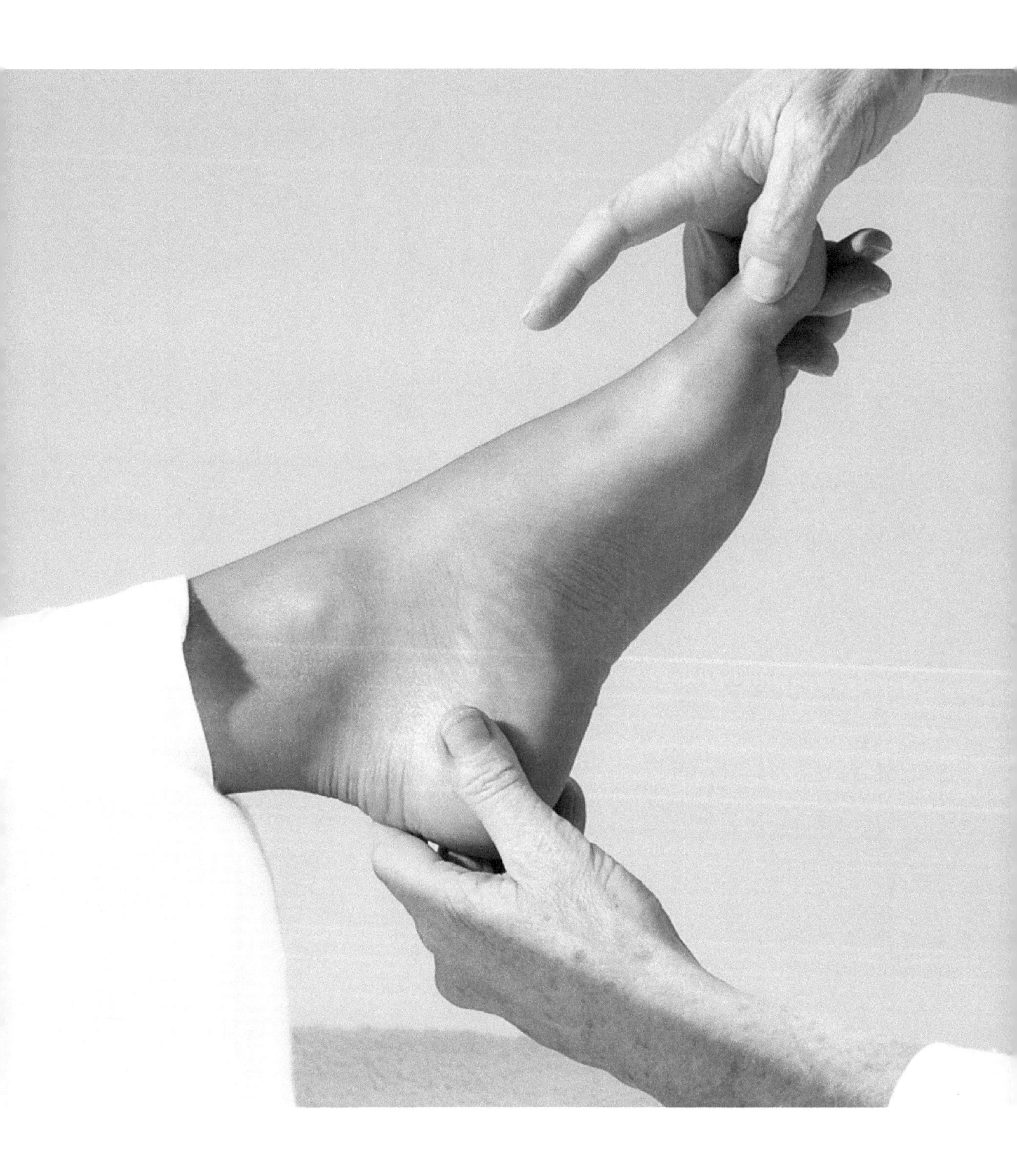

Section 3

REFLEXOLOGY LYMPH DRAINAGE

Chapter 6
Step by Step Guide to Reflexology Lymph Drainage

Expectation

So far in this book you have read about my reflexology journey and the creation of RLD from first principles. To enable you to implement the original protocol, each step is illustrated and has a detailed description of the reflex, how to find it on the feet, and how to work each move sequentially.

Once you have mastered and understood the original protocol, learn how to integrate RLD into your practice for clients with a wide variety of different presenting conditions.

At the end of this chapter there is a summary of the original RLD sequence for unilateral secondary lymphoedema of the arm.

Introduction

As reflexologists we all find our own unique way of working. This develops through life experiences, our training, clinical practice and other influencing factors. In reflexology there will always be things you like and things you don't! A "Ted" lesson that has stayed with me was "once you start don't let go" and I have worked this way ever since. I always prefer treatment to flow continuously, rather than to feel disjointed if contact with the foot is broken. As a result of this RLD flows gently with a smooth transition from one step of the sequence to the next. It is a fluent, gentle and effective treatment to give and receive.

The RLD protocol was formalised for part of the NHS ethics application, as previously explained, because the ethics committee require the exact details of the proposed intervention. The following sequence is the original protocol and it has been used in all RLD research to date to achieve the remarkable results (see Chapter 9 on page 167).

MLD and SLD are the foundation on which RLD was created by using the anatomical reflection theory to reflect these first principles onto the reflexes of the feet. The aim was to create a relaxing and enjoyable reflexology treatment able to cause an effect on the lymphatic drainage and reduce lymphoedema swelling.

Note: Coincidentally, years later when I visited China, every foot reflexology treatment I received was given this way, nurturing and working one foot at a time, deeply and completely before starting the other foot. This makes perfect sense to me and there was a familiarity to it, going the full circle, as Ted first learnt reflexology in China (see Chapter 11 on page 216).

Recap of the lymph journey: This begins when it enters the initial lymphatics, and moves away from the cells in lymph vessels towards the lymph nodes where it is filtered before entering larger lymph vessels. These eventually converge into lymphatic ducts which return the fluid to the blood circulation via the subclavian vein (see Chapter 3 on page 60).

Previously in Chapter 3 of this book I explained how space needs to be created for lymph to enter the system from the interstitial spaces. This is different to massage, which increases the circulation by encouraging movement in a continuous two-way systemic cycle (oxygenated arterial blood flow and de-oxygenated venous return). The lymph journey begins when interstitial fluid enters the initial lymphatic vessels and ends at the subclavian vein.

To understand the first principles of RLD, it helps to look at this lymph journey in reverse because this is how to effect a change.

- Subclavian vein (SCV) - drains filtered lymph back to the blood circulation
- Lymphatic ducts - drain into the subclavian vein
- Thoracic duct - transports lymph from the abdomen and legs up the body
- Cisterna chyli - stores lymph and empties into the thoracic duct
- Larger lymph vessels - transports filtered lymph away from the nodes
- Lymph nodes - filters lymph from smaller vessels
- Smaller vessels - transports lymph towards the nodes
- Initial lymphatics - collects fluid from interstitial spaces

Decide where to begin - choose the foot carefully!

Empty space must first be created to cause an effect on the drainage function and reduce the swelling by encouraging the excess fluid into the lymphatic system from the interstitial spaces. For this to happen RLD (like MLD & SLD) needs to drain away the lymph that is already in the system and move it to return towards the blood circulation. Think of the subclavian vein as the drain, the exit channel for lymph to leave the system and re-enter the blood flow. As this happens space is created at the other end, the initial lymphatics, for excess interstitial fluid to enter the lymphatic system.

Remember that MLD and SLD begin by working to clear the normal side of the body, to create a space so the lymph has somewhere to go before working on the swollen side. These moves are then repeated on the normal side again to end the treatment. Therefore, RLD starts with the foot that corresponds to the normal arm, before working on the foot on the side of the swollen arm. Repeat the sequence again on the first foot, and thus work 3 feet for clients with unilateral secondary lymphoedema of the arm.

For lymphoedema of the left arm start with the right foot

- Right foot
- Left foot
- Right foot

For lymphoedema of the right arm start with the left foot

- Left foot
- Right foot
- Left foot

RLD flows sequentially, and each reflex has a role in stimulating the drainage function. Here's how it's done, in a comprehensive, illustrated step by step guide to the RLD reflexes and how to work them in consecutive order.

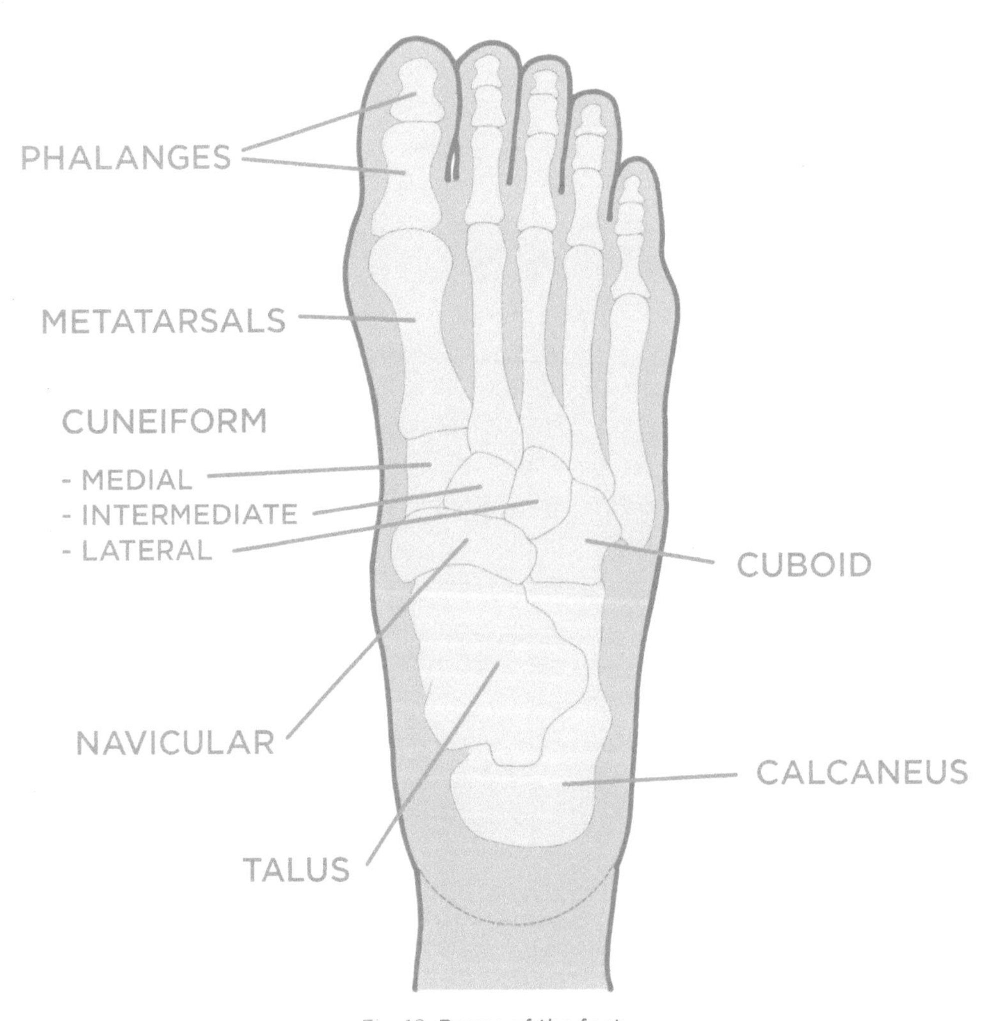

Fig. 18: **Bones of the feet**

RLD reflexes - step by step

Step 1: The diaphragm

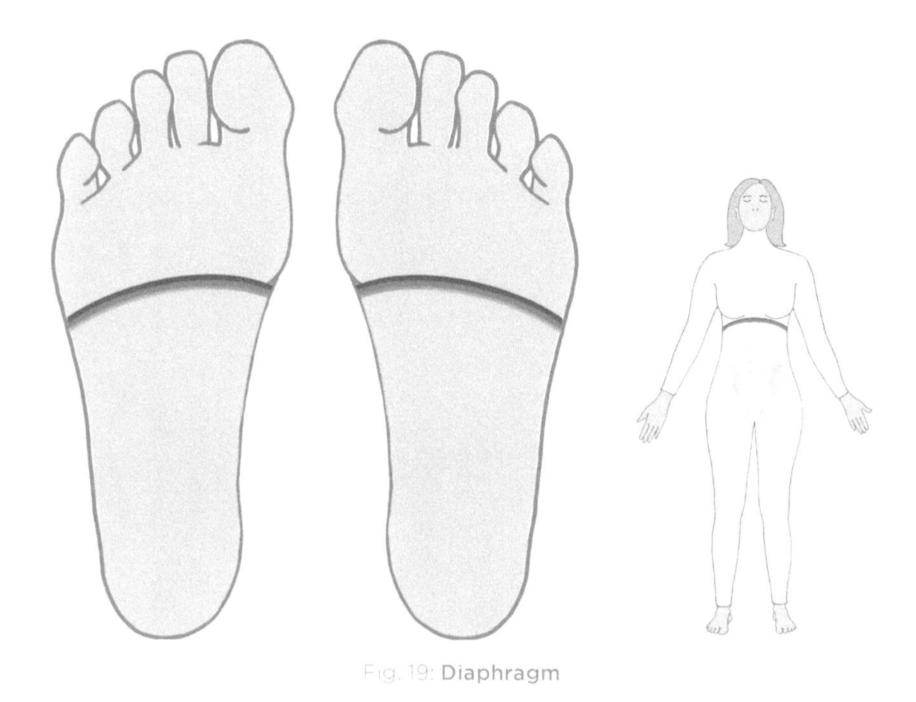

Fig. 19: **Diaphragm**

In MLD & SLD the action of the deep diaphragmatic breathing helps the lymph travel up the body in the thoracic duct.

Start at the lateral edge of the foot, and thumb walk across the diaphragm reflex 5 times. Work from the lateral edge of the plantar to medial edge and count that as one (1), change hands and work medial to lateral (2), finishing the fifth time at the medial edge of the foot, in position for the next move.

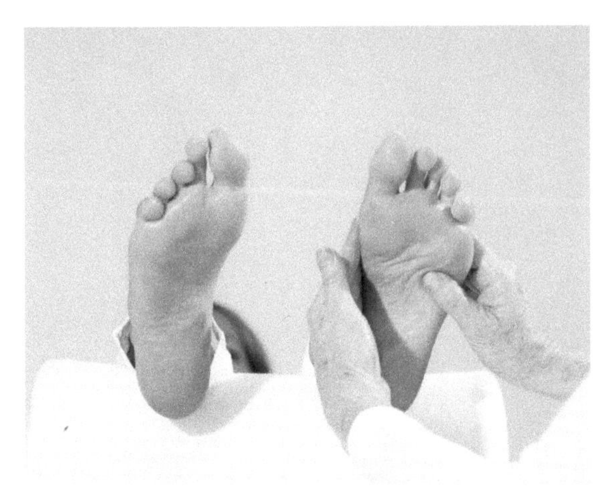

1: Work from the lateral edge of the plantar to medial edge and count that as one

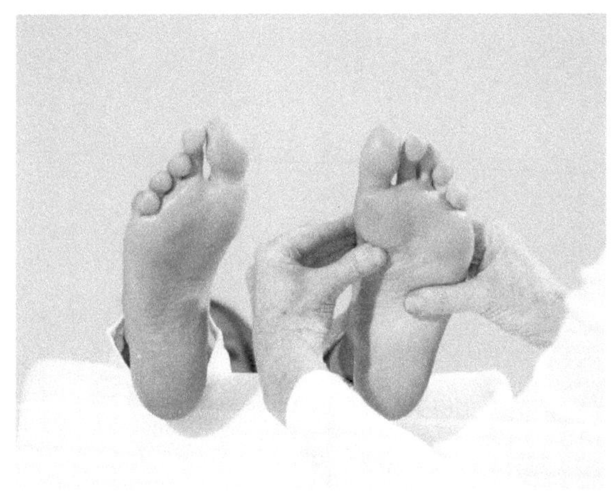

2: Change hands and work medial to lateral

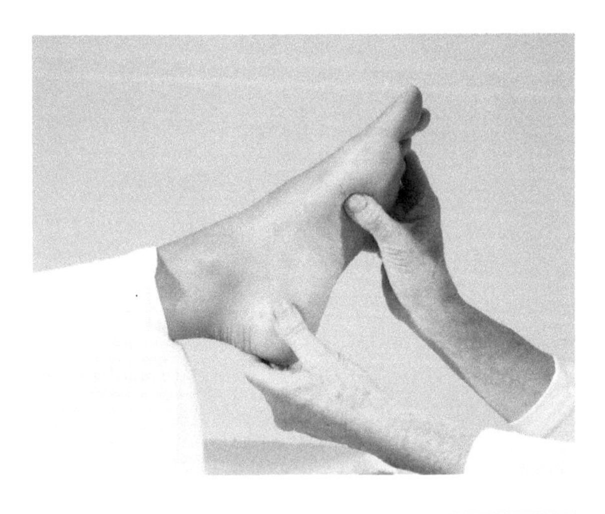

3: Finishing the fifth time at the medial edge of the foot

Step 2: Spinal cord, cisterna chyli, thoracic duct and subclavian vein

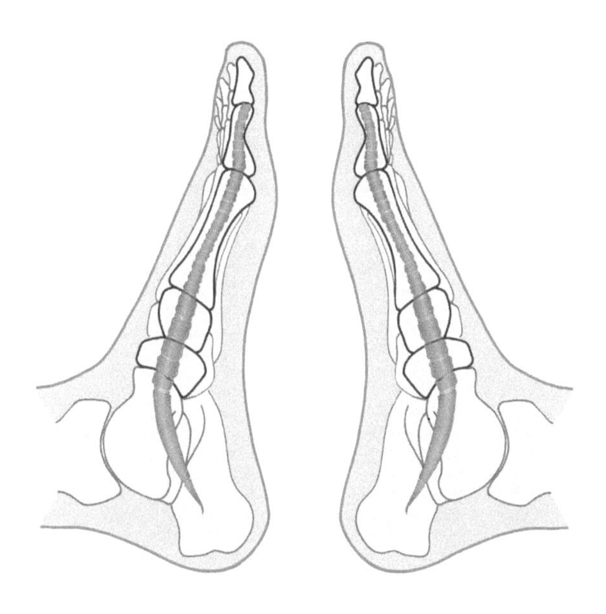

Fig. 20: **Spine reflex**

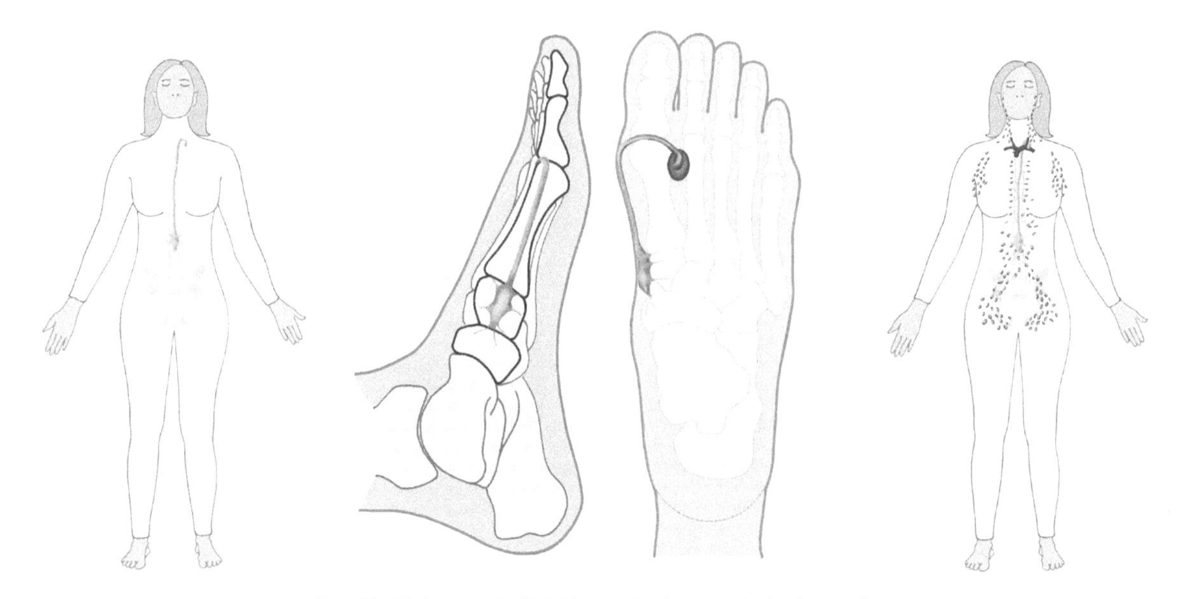

Fig. 21: **Cisterna chyli & thoracic duct, subclavian vein**

Step 2a: Spinal cord

Hold the big toe and support the foot with the free hand.

To work the spinal cord reflex, thumb walk down along the medial edge of the first phalange and metatarsal bone and beyond to the head of the navicular bone (third lumbar vertebra reflex).

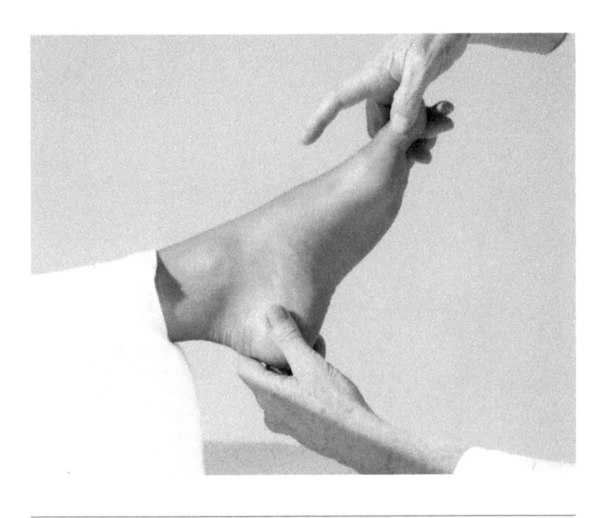

1: Hold the big toe and support the foot with the free hand. Thumb walk down along the medial edge of the first phalange

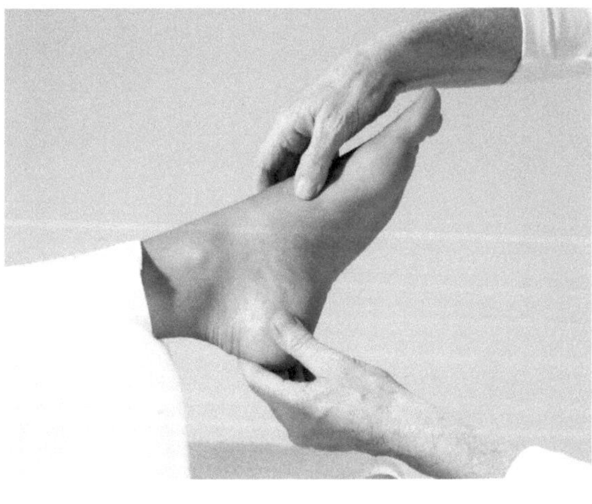

2: Continue along the medial edge of the metatarsal bone

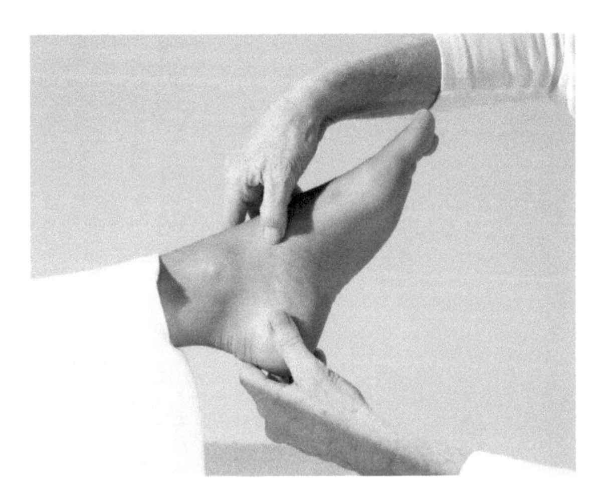

3: To the head of the navicular bone (third lumbar vertebra reflex)

Step 2b (i): Cisterna chyli

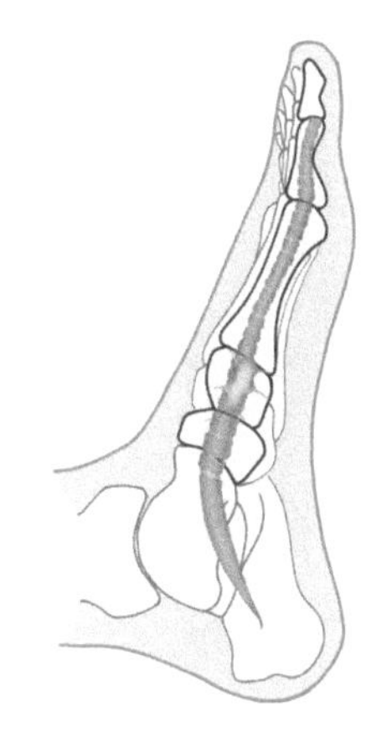

Fig. 22: Cisterna chyli reflex

The cisterna chyli reflex is on the medial edge of the cuneiform bone.

Swap hands and replace the working thumb of 2a with the other thumb (see photos). Slide off the head of the navicular onto the medial edge of the cuneiform bone into the cisterna chyli reflex. Pause briefly and press gently before moving to the thoracic duct reflex.

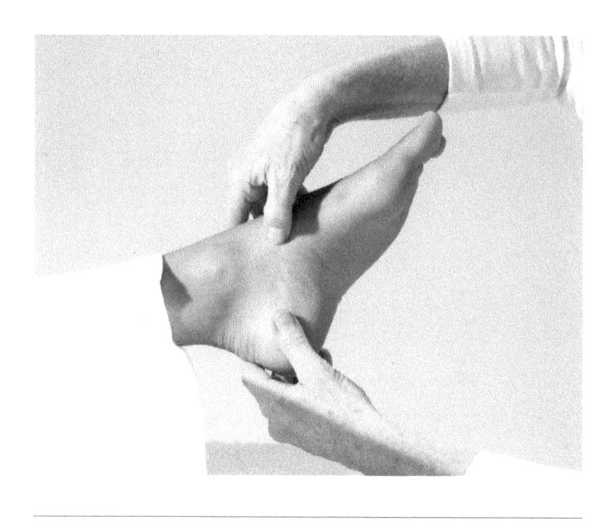

4: Swap hands and replace the working thumb of 2a with the other thumb

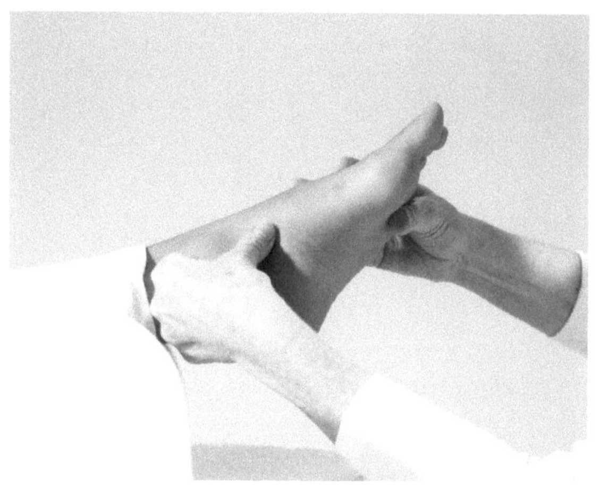

5: Slide off the head of the navicular onto the medial edge of the cuneiform bone into the cisterna chyli reflex

Note: In some cases the cisterna chyli reflex is visibly puffy, more so on the left foot. Remember the left side of the lymphatic system drains three quarters of the body.

Step 2b (ii): Thoracic duct

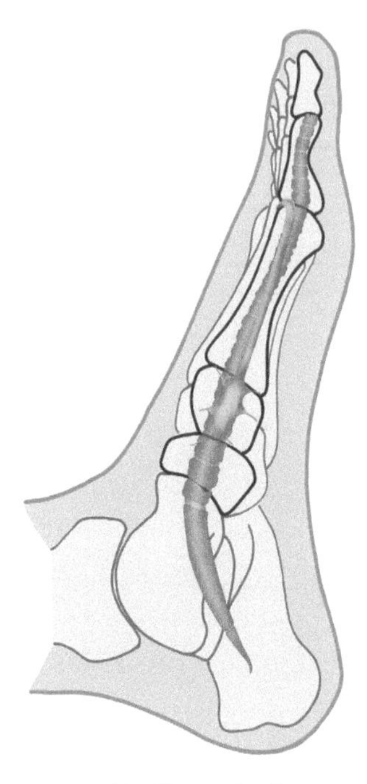

Fig. 23: **Thoracic duct**

> Lymph collects in the cisterna chyli, before being transported up the body in the thoracic duct and returned to the circulation via the left subclavian vein

Thumb walk up the thoracic duct reflex along the medial edge of the first metatarsal bone.

At the base of the big toe, change from thumb to index finger and slide across the dorsal base of the big toe, and down between the first two metatarsals to the subclavian vein reflex.

Repeat this sequence 3 times.

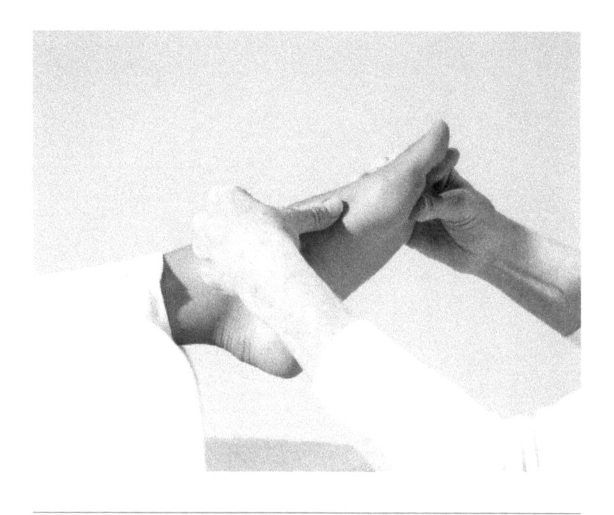

6: Thumb walk up the thoracic duct reflex along the medial edge of the first metatarsal bone.

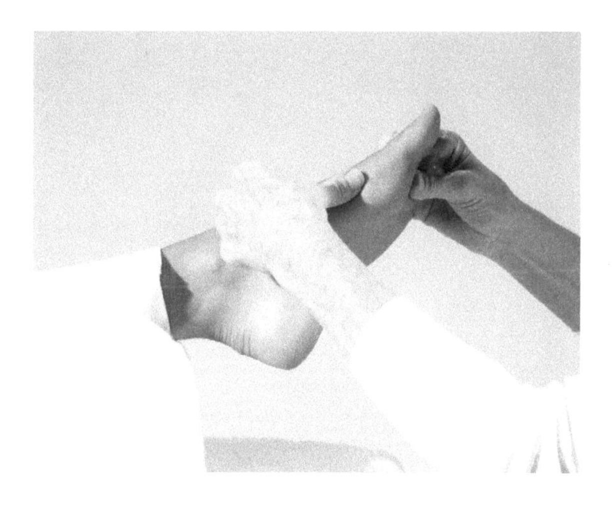

7: To the first metatarsophalangeal joint

Step 2b (iii): Subclavian vein

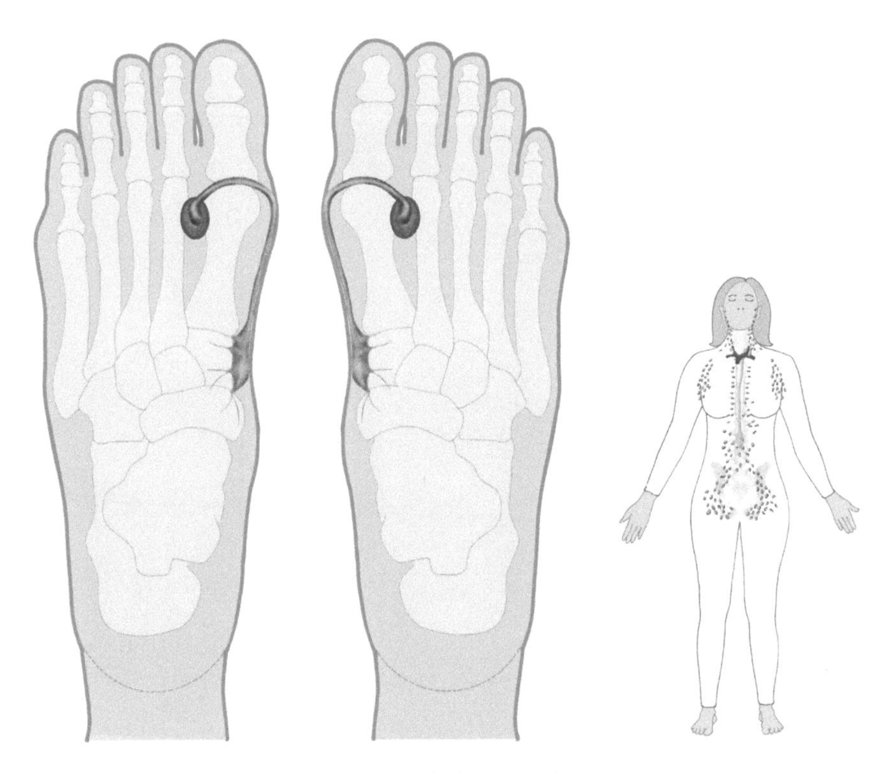

Fig. 24: **Subclavian vein**

The subclavian vein reflex is located on the dorsal between the first and second metatarsal. To find this reflex, use the pad of the index finger and gently slide down between the first and second metatarsals, until you find an obvious dip.

Once the subclavian vein is open lymph can begin to flow.

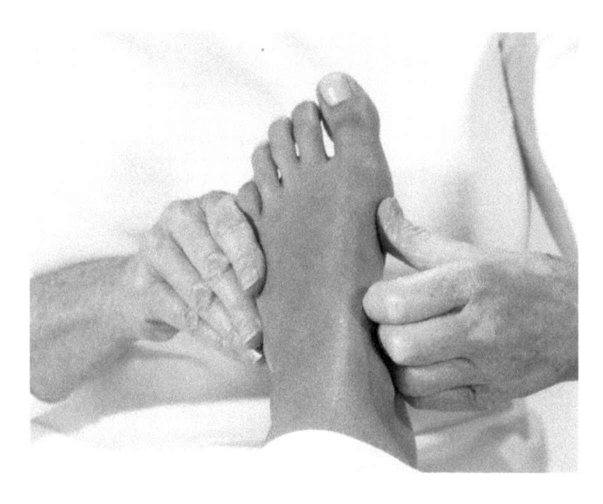

8: At the base of the big toe, change from thumb to index finger

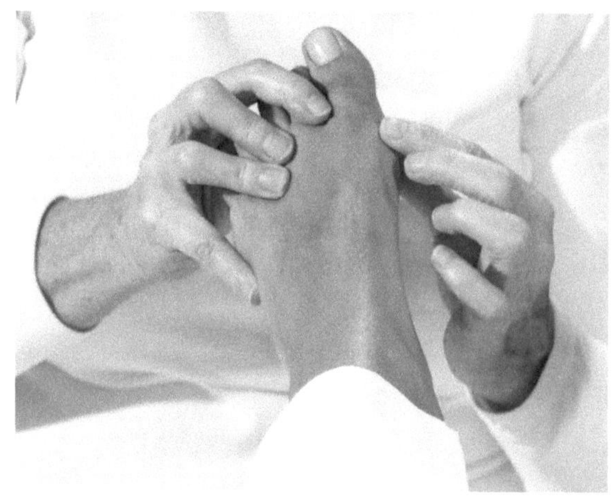

9: Slide across the dorsal base of the big toe

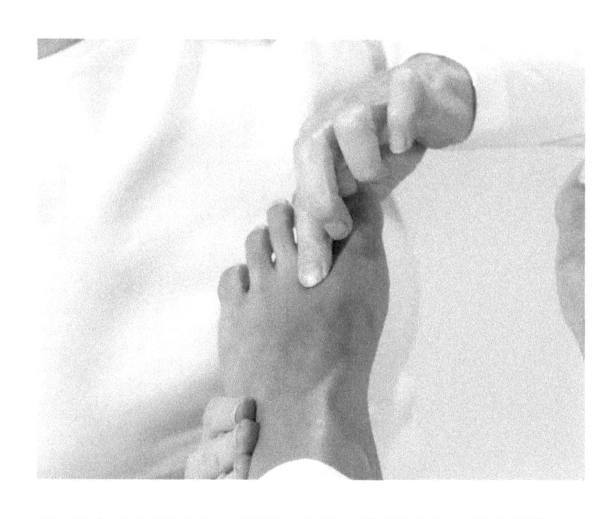

10: Down between the first two metatarsals to the subclavian vein reflex

Steps 2a & 2b are one move – "down, up & in"

- Thumb walk down the spinal cord reflex to the head of the navicular bone and swap thumbs
- Slide into the cisterna chyli reflex, press gently on the medial edge of the cuneiform bone
- Thumb walk up the thoracic duct along the medial edge of the first metatarsal
- Swap to index finger to slide across the dorsal base of big toe into the subclavian vein reflex
- Repeat 3 times

Step 3: Cervical lymph nodes, Upper trapezius and Back of the underarm

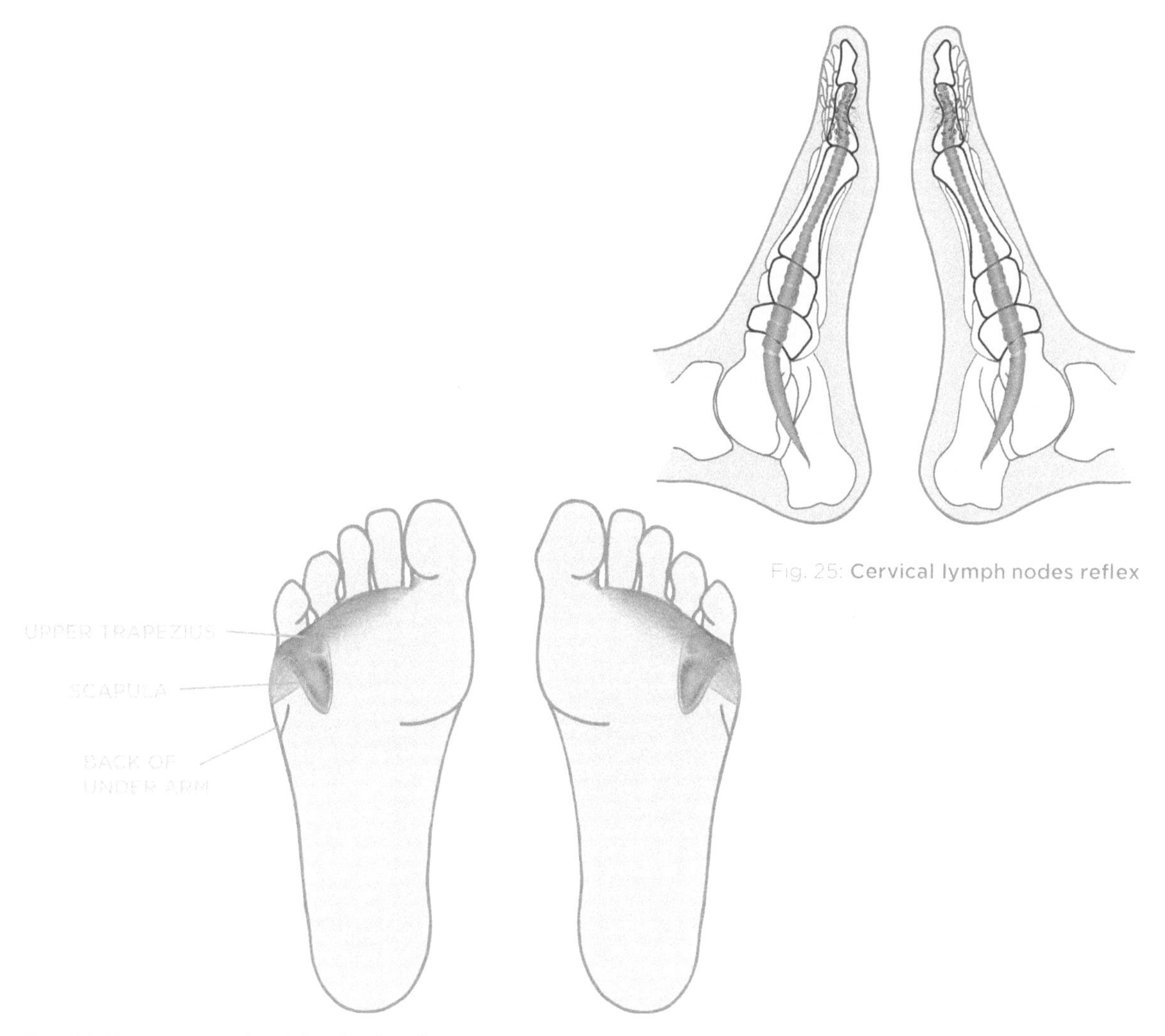

Fig. 25: Cervical lymph nodes reflex

Fig. 26: Upper trapezius & back of underarm

NOTE: In SLD, this move is to open up at the neck by gently working the lymph nodes at the sides of the neck to stimulate lymph movement and drainage at the neck.

Step 3a: Cervical lymph nodes

Work the cervical lymph nodes reflex, which is on the medial edge of the first phalange (see Fig. 25). Stimulate this reflex with a circular movement of the skin against the surface of the bone.

Thumb walk around the back of the neck reflex on the plantar of the big toe.

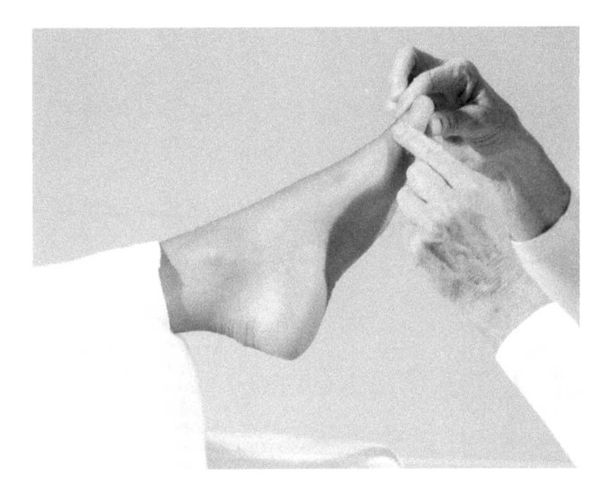

1: Stimulate the cervical lymph nodes reflex with a circular movement of the skin against the surface of the bone

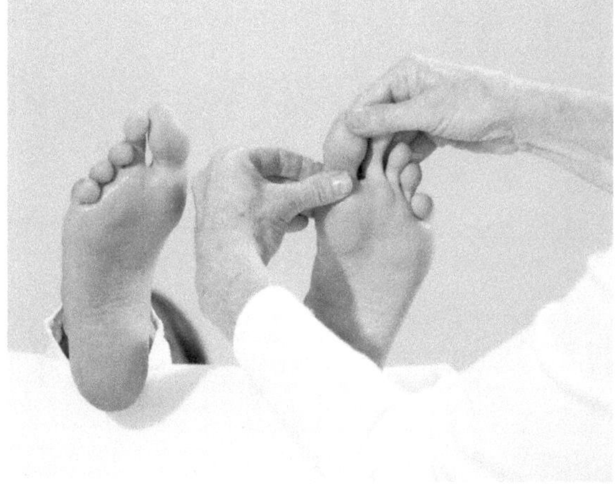

2: Thumb walk around the back of the neck reflex on the plantar of the big toe

NOTE: Observe the client for signs of swallowing. They may experience an increase of saliva in the mouth.

3b (i) & 3b (ii): Upper trapezius, and Back of the underarm

Circle along the upper trapezius reflex as far as the fourth toe. Work down around the scapula reflex to the lateral edge of the foot to the reflex area for the back of the underarm (see Fig. 26).

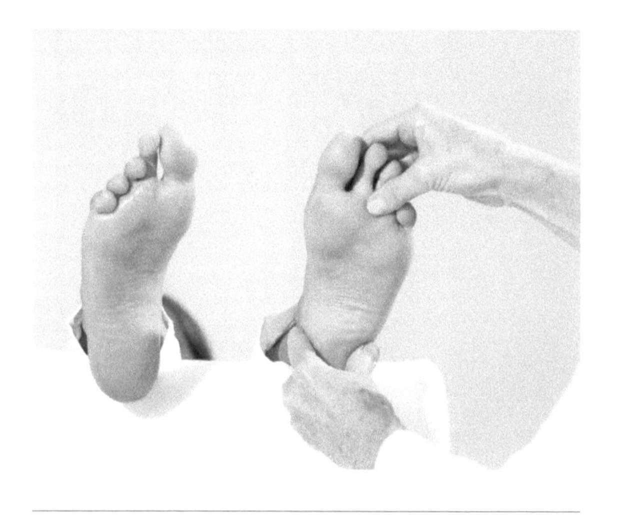

3: Circle along the upper trapezius reflex as far as the fourth toe

4: Work down around the scapula reflex

Turn around and return from lateral to medial. Use the thumb to push back up around the scapula and thumb walk back along the upper trapezius as far as the second toe. Rotate the working hand 90 degrees, keep contact with the thumb at the plantar base of the second toe and place the index finger of the working hand on the dorsal, between the first and second metatarsals, and slide it down into the subclavian vein reflex.

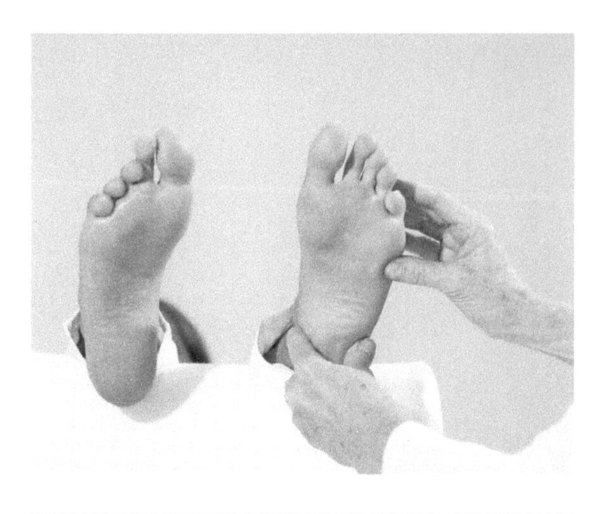

5: To the lateral edge of the foot to the reflex area for the back of the underarm

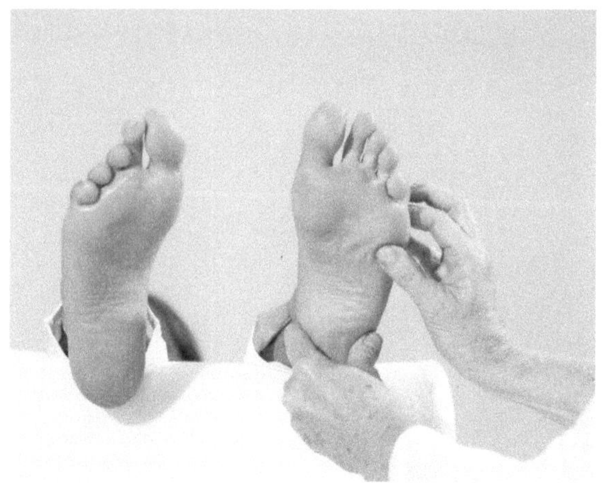

6: Turn around and return from lateral to medial. Use the thumb to push back up around the scapula

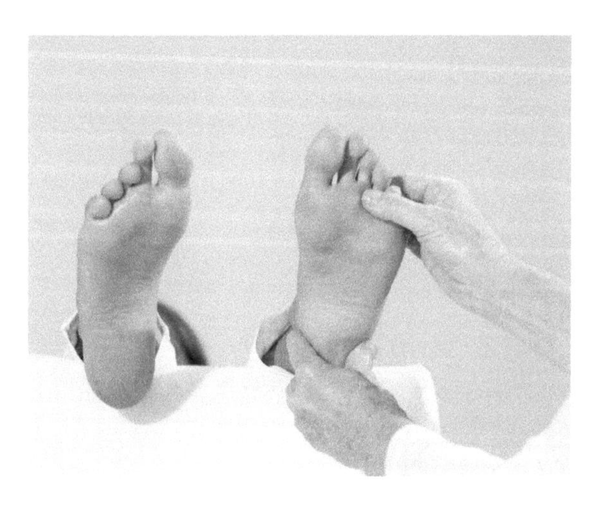

7: Thumb walk back along the upper trapezius as far as the second toe

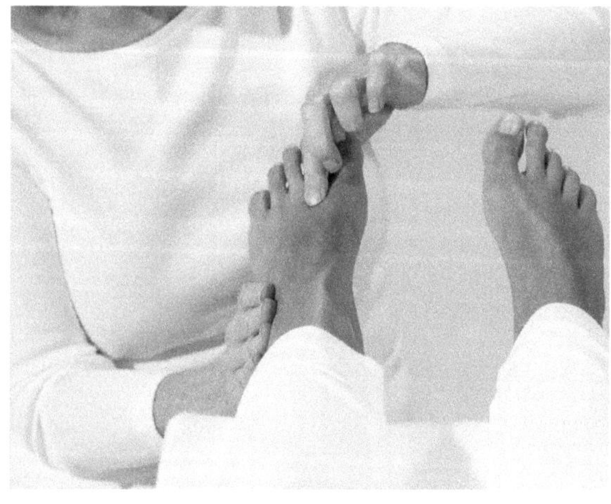

8: Rotate the working hand 90 degrees, keep contact with the thumb at the plantar base of the second toe and place the index finger of the working hand on the dorsal, slide it down into the subclavian vein reflex

Summary of 3a & 3b as one move:

- Gently circle the cervical lymph node
- Work around the back of the neck
- Circle along the upper trapezius
- Down around the scapula to the back of underarm
- Reverse and return to the subclavian vein
- Back up around the scapula
- Thumb walk back along the upper trapezius as far as the second toe, rotate working hand, and with the index finger slide into the subclavian vein reflex

Repeat 3a & 3b together 3 times.

Finish at the subclavian vein, in the correct position to continue with the dorsal upper lymph reflexes.

Step 4: Upper lymph reflexes (dorsal)

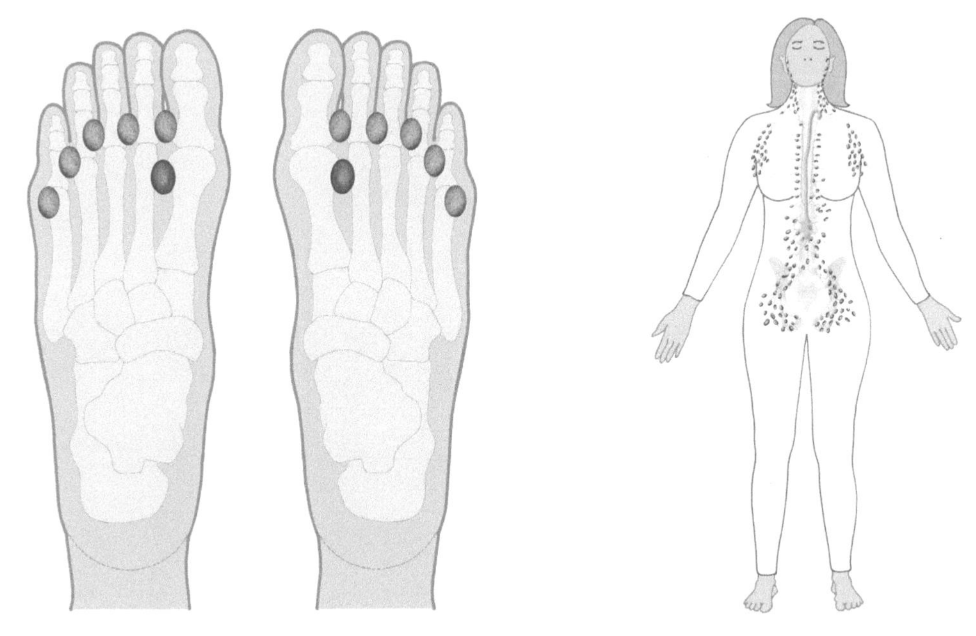

Fig. 27: **Upper lymph**

Upper lymph reflexes of steps 4, 5 & 6 are worked from the medial to lateral and back into the subclavian vein. Repeat 3 times.

Slide towards the toes from the subclavian vein reflex into the first of the upper lymph reflexes, using light contact to avoid dragging up against the flow of lymph. Work from medial to lateral, keep the working hand high and use a circular movement in each upper lymph reflex. Transition smoothly between each of the five upper lymph reflexes, which include the axilla (underarm) reflex, which is located under the distal head of the fifth metatarsal.

Reverse these steps to return from lateral to medial and back into the subclavian vein.

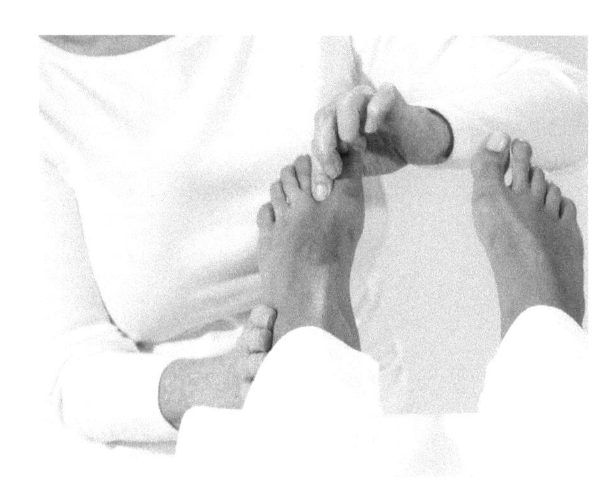

1: Slide towards the toes from the subclavian vein reflex into the first of the upper lymph reflexes

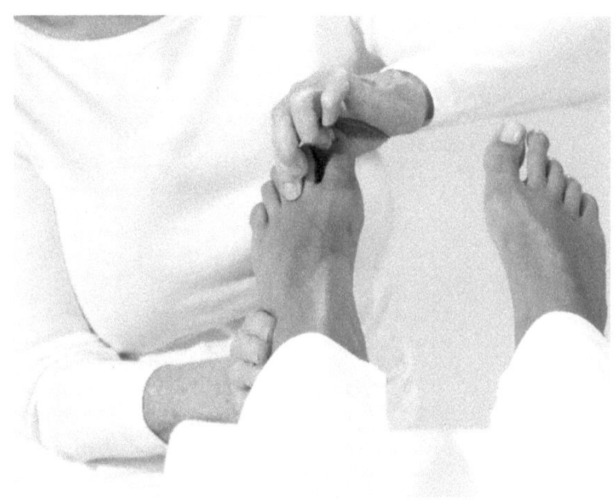

2: Work from medial to lateral, keep the working hand high and use a circular movement in each upper lymph reflex

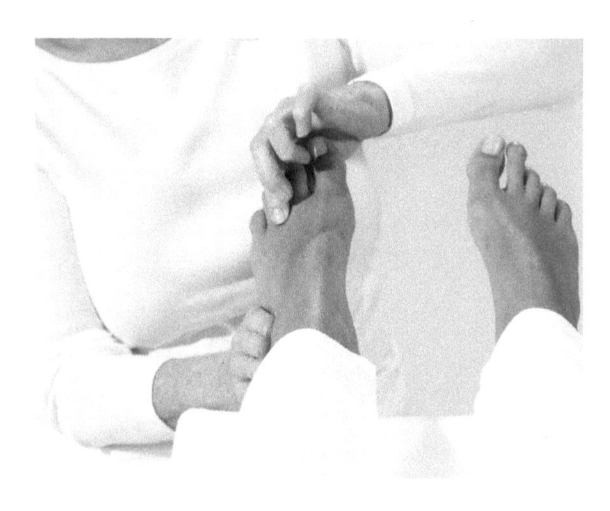

3: Transition smoothly between each of the upper lymph reflexes

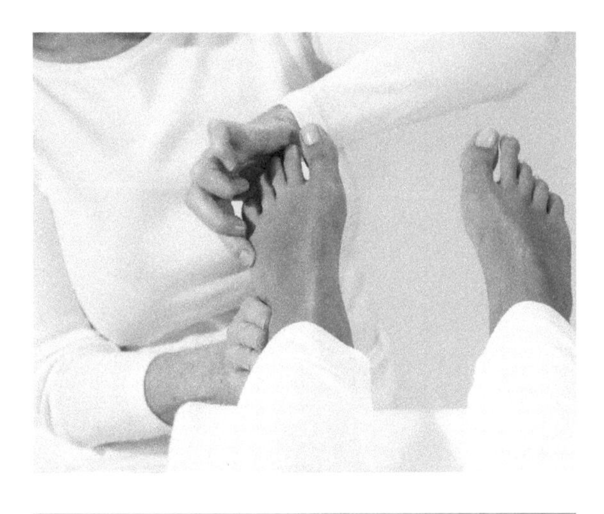

4: Include the axilla (underarm) reflex just below the distal head of the fifth metatarsal

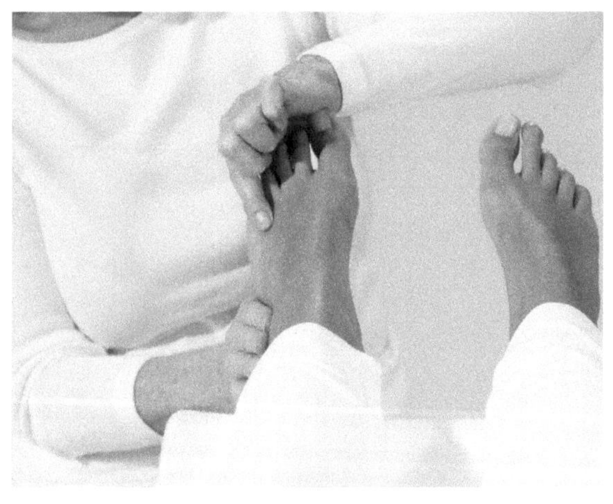

5: Circle back across the upper lymph reflexes from lateral to medial

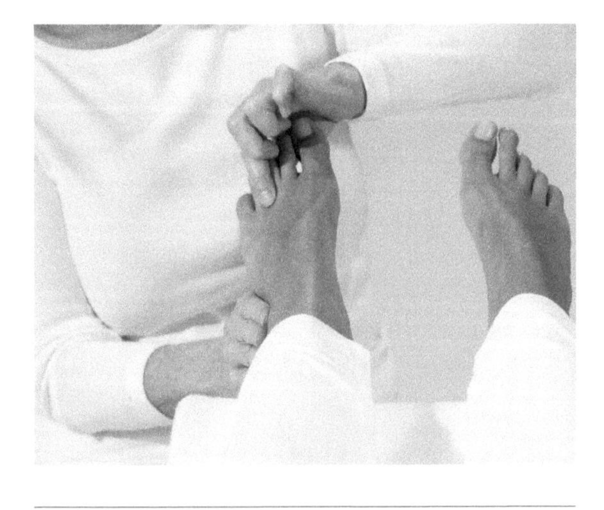

6: Keep the working hand high

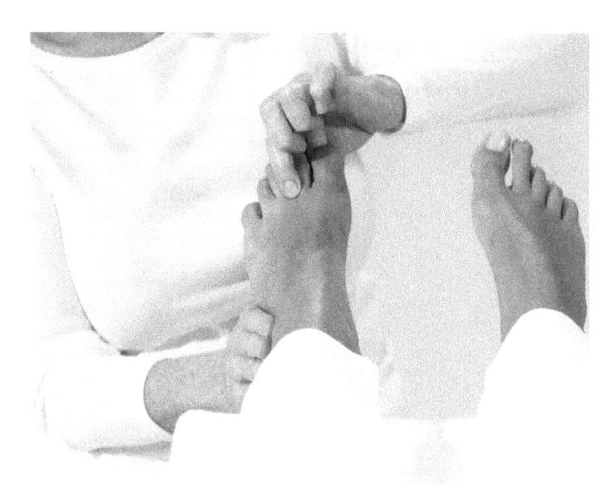

7: Circle in each upper lymph reflex

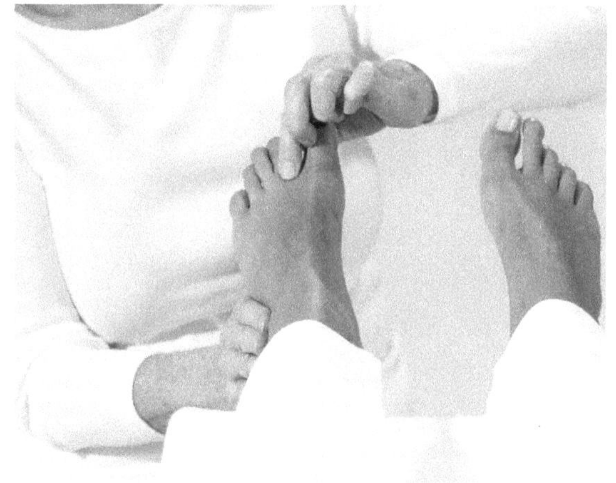

8: Keep contact and transition smoothly between each reflex

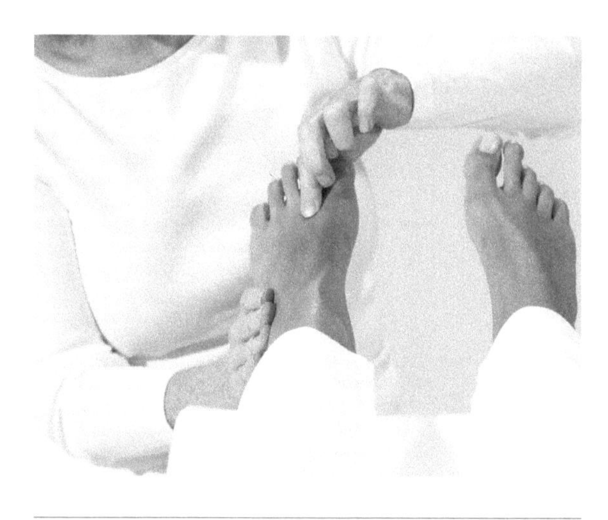

9: Finish at the subclavian vein

Step 5: Upper lymph to lateral shoulder reflex - deltoid muscle

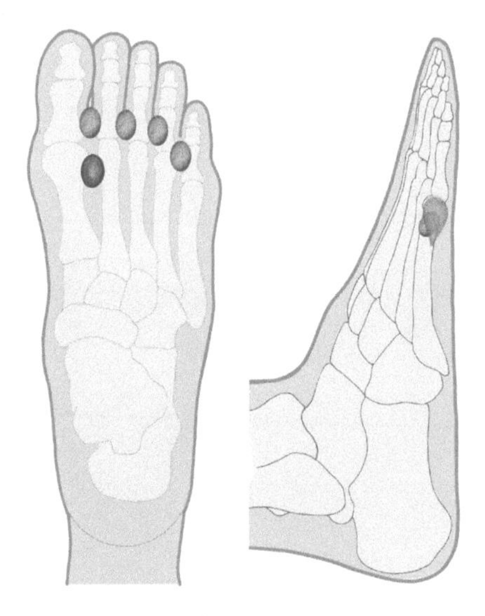

Fig. 28: **Lateral shoulder - deltoid reflex**

From the subclavian vein reflex, circle across the upper lymph reflexes as before (see step 4) to the lateral edge of the foot, to the pad of soft tissue, the deltoid muscle reflex (or lateral shoulder). Gently work the reflex area, either thumb walking or knuckling, and remember it is the soft tissue of the lateral shoulder, and not deep in the shoulder joint.

Circle back across the upper lymph reflexes from lateral to medial to the subclavian vein.

Repeat 3 times, across from medial to lateral to the shoulder and back to the subclavian vein.

NOTE: This area is worked to clear any lymphoedema congestion that may have built up above the compression garment. It also helps to clear the space for the rest of the arm to drain.

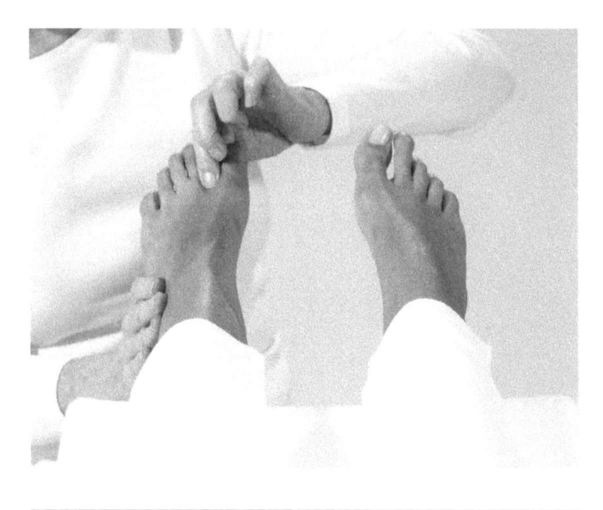

1: Slide towards the toes from the subclavian vein reflex into the first of the upper lymph reflexes

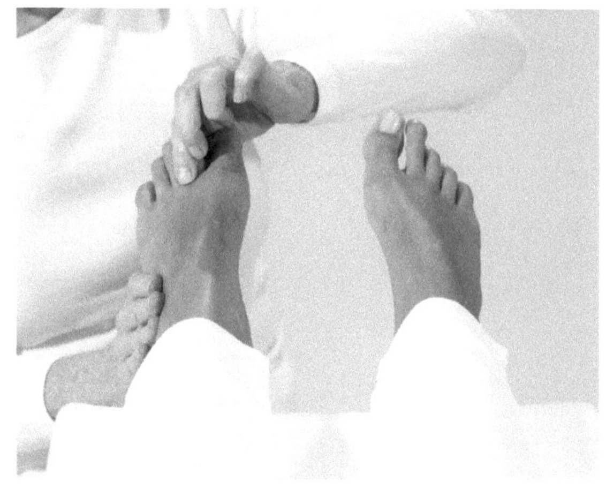

2: Work from medial to lateral, keep the working hand high and use a circular movement in each upper lymph reflex

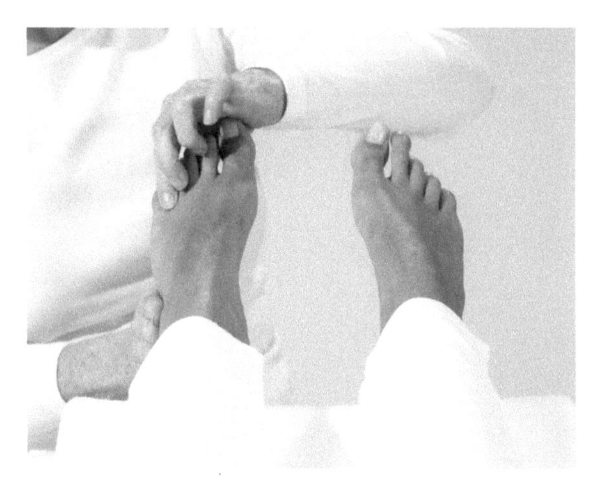

3: Transition smoothly between each of the upper lymph reflexes

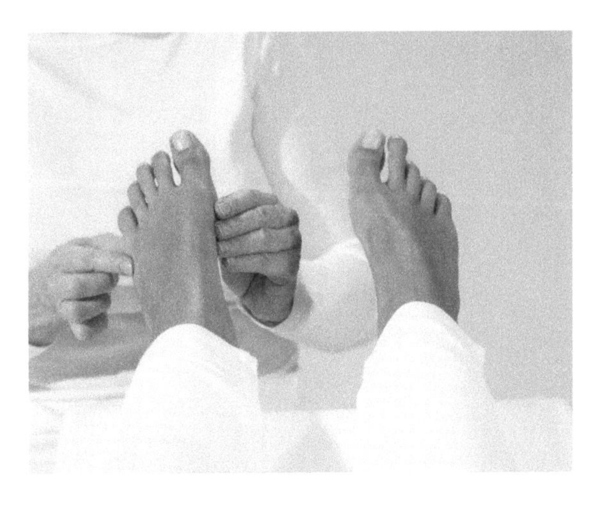

4: To the lateral edge of the foot, to the pad of soft tissue of the deltoid muscle reflex of the lateral shoulder

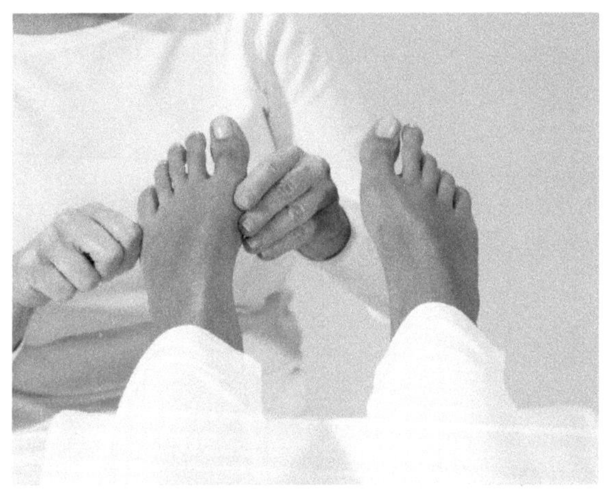

5: Gently work the lateral shoulder either thumb walking or knuckling

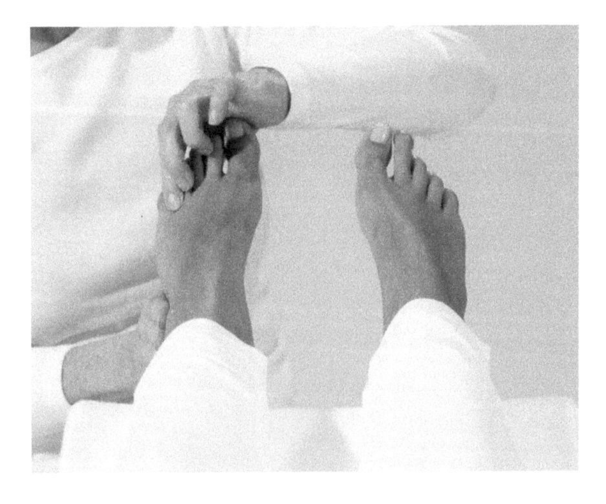

6: Circle back across the upper lymph reflexes from lateral to medial

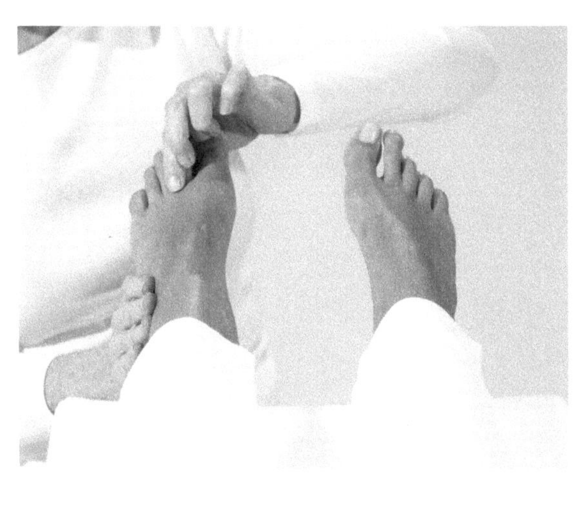

7: Keep the working hand high

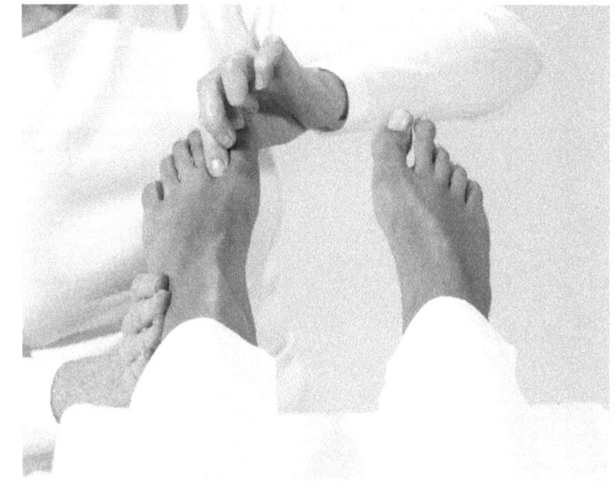

8: Keep contact and transition smoothly between circling in each reflex

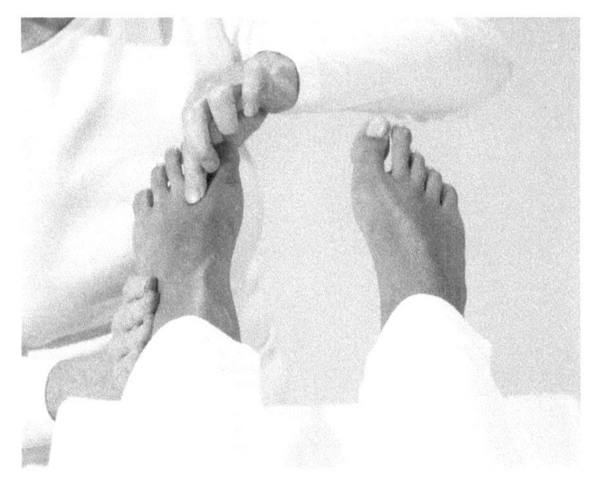

9: Into the subclavian vein

Step 6: Upper lymph to underarm (pump) – Axillary lymph nodes

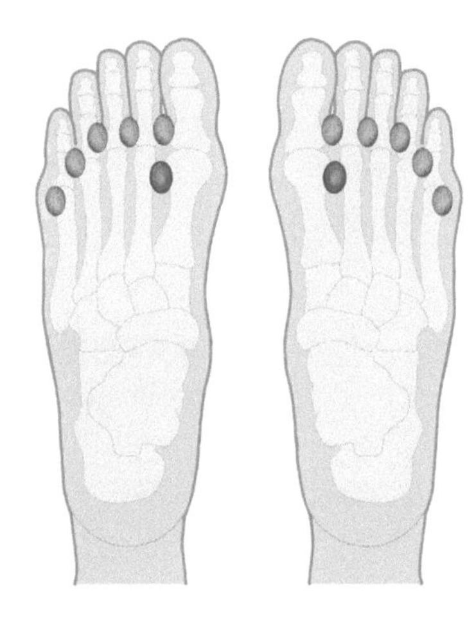

Fig. 29: **Upper lymph to underarm reflexes**

NOTE: In SLD, a pumping action under the arm is to help encourage the lymph nodes to empty, which creates space, a vacuum to encourage interstitial fluid to enter the system.

From the subclavian vein reflex, circle across the upper lymph reflexes as before (see step 4) to the lateral edge of the foot.

At the fifth upper lymph reflex (axilla/underarm), hook up and under the distal head of the fifth metatarsal with the pad of the index or middle finger and gently pump the reflex 3 times.

Circle back across the upper lymph reflexes from lateral to medial to the subclavian vein.

Repeat 3 times from medial to lateral: pump under the arm and return back from lateral to medial to the subclavian vein.

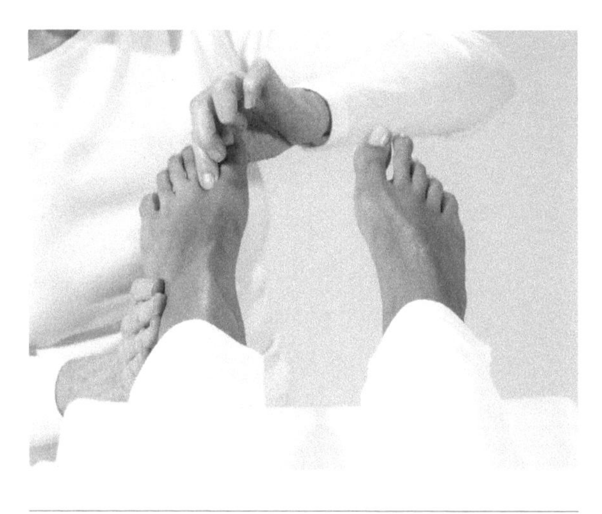

1: Slide towards the toes from the subclavian vein reflex into the first of the upper lymph reflexes

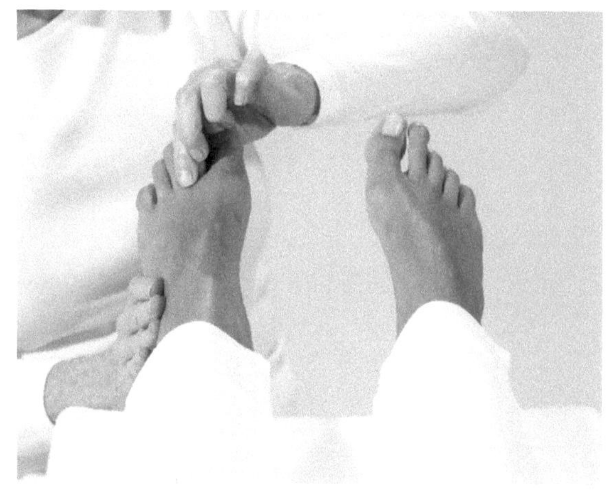

2: Work from medial to lateral, keep the working hand high and use a circular movement in each upper lymph reflex

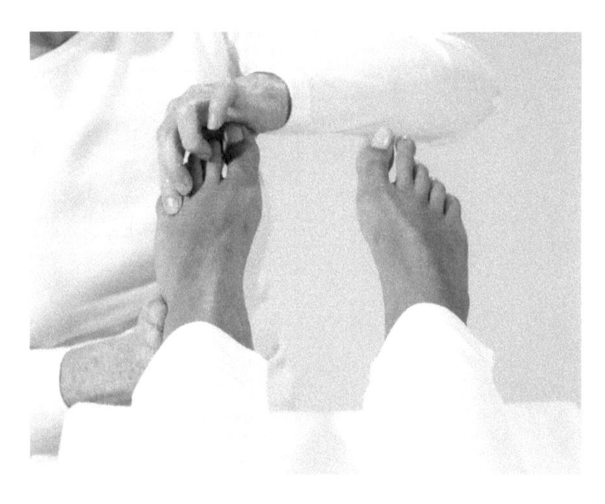

3: Transition smoothly between each of the five upper lymph reflexes

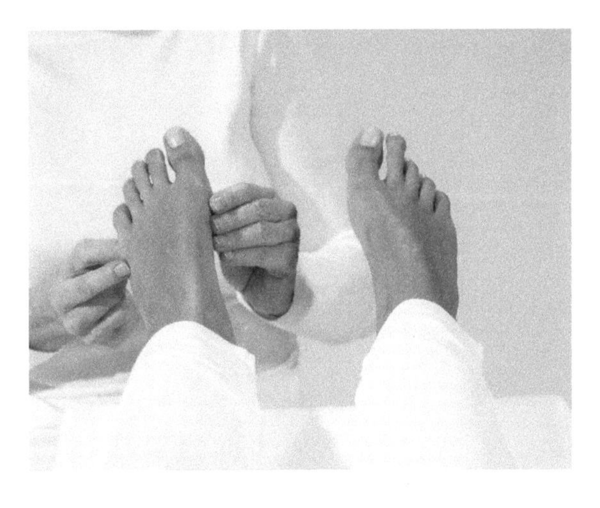

4: To the axilla

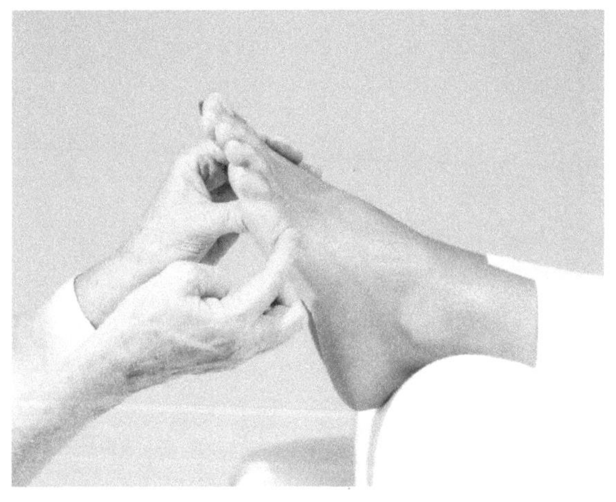

5: Gently pump underarm reflex 3 times.

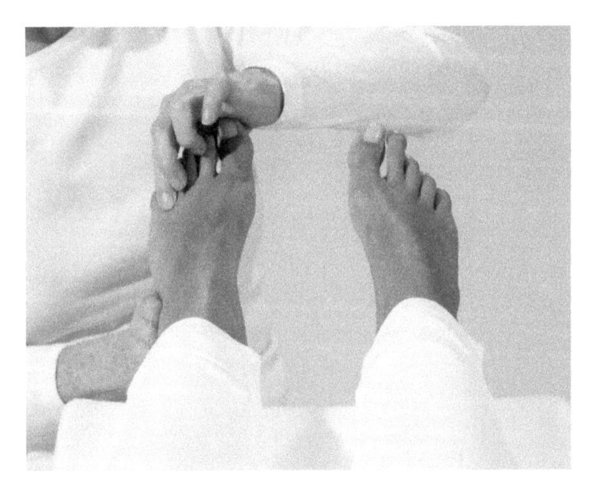

6: Reverse this and circle back across the upper lymph reflexes

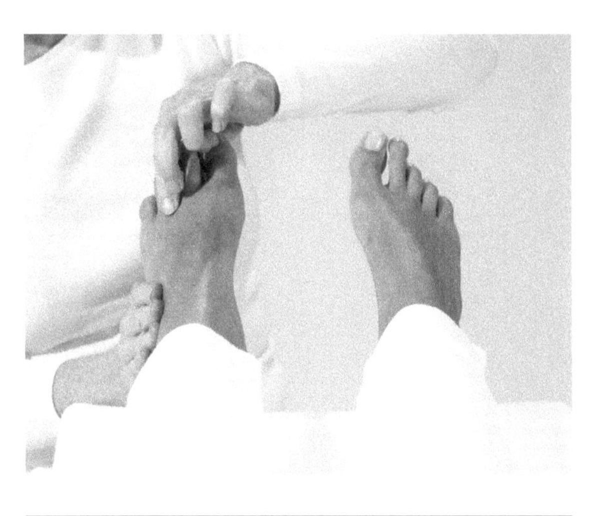

7: Keep contact and transition smoothly between each upper lymph reflex

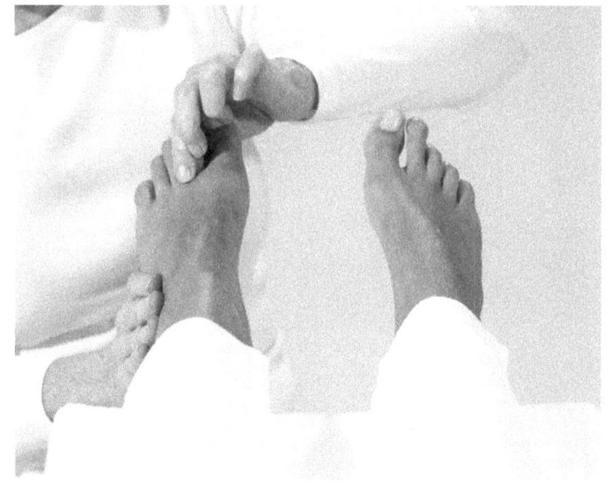

8: From lateral to medial as before

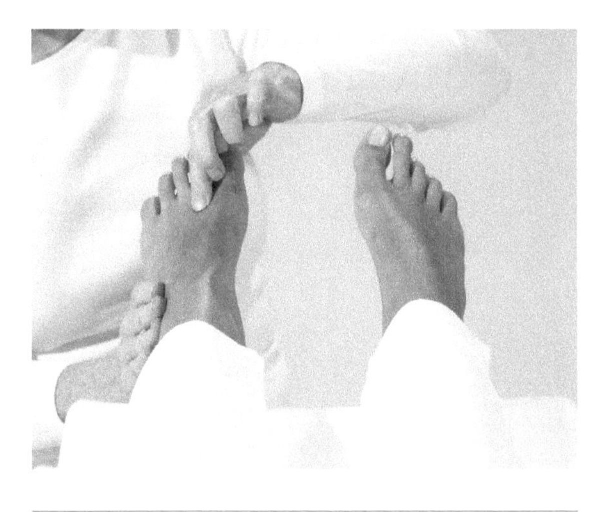

9: Return the lymph to the subclavian vein

Step 7: Lower lymph

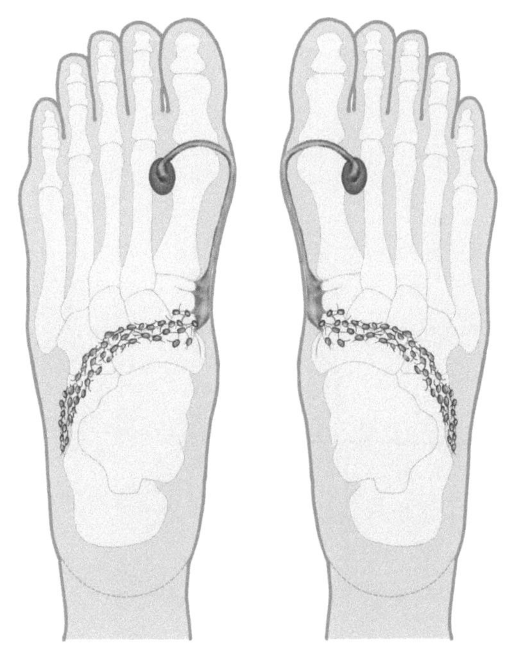

Fig. 30: **Lower lymphatic reflexes (medial to lateral)**

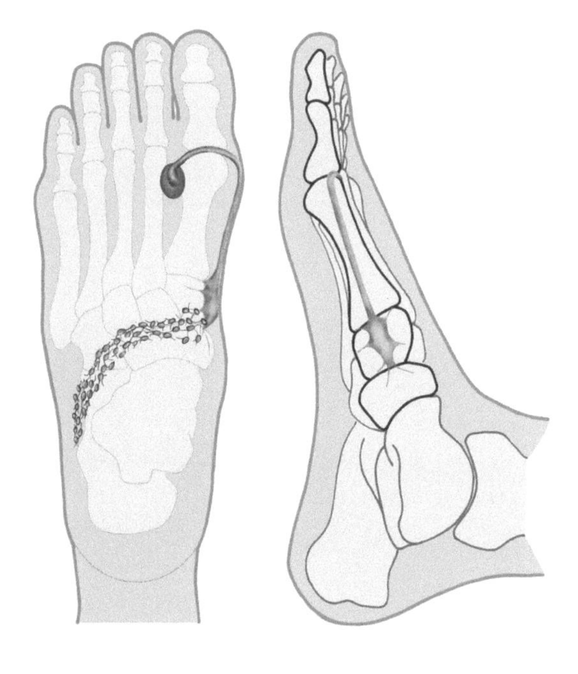

Fig. 31: **Lower lymph (lateral to medial) thoracic duct & subclavian vein**

NOTE: Anatomical reflection: Lower lymphatic reflexes are situated at the articulation of dorsiflexion where the ankle flexes. To find the reflex, place one hand on the plantar and slightly dorsiflex the foot. Use your other hand to locate and work across the lower lymph, inguinal reflex area.

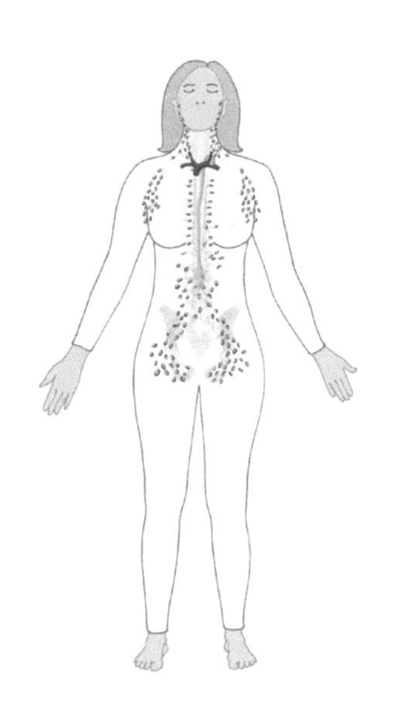

7a: Lower lymphatic reflexes (medial to lateral)

With both hands, use a light effleurage to sweep down over the dorsal and around the ankle to the lower lymph reflex.

Support the foot with the hand on the lateral edge, and with the index and middle finger of the free hand hook/finger walk across the lower lymph reflexes from medial to lateral.

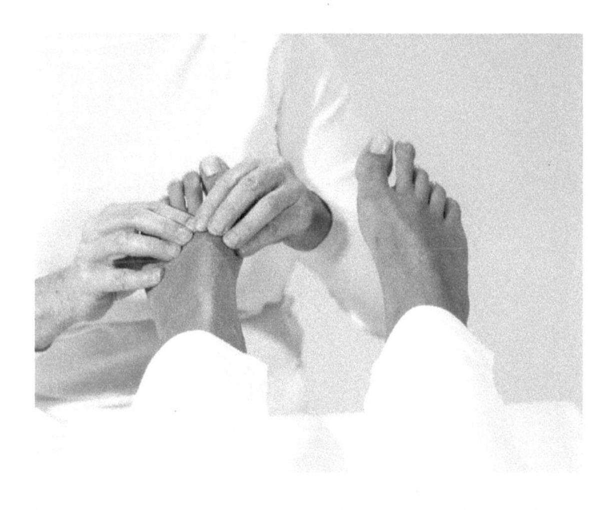

1: With both hands, use a light effleurage to sweep down over the dorsal

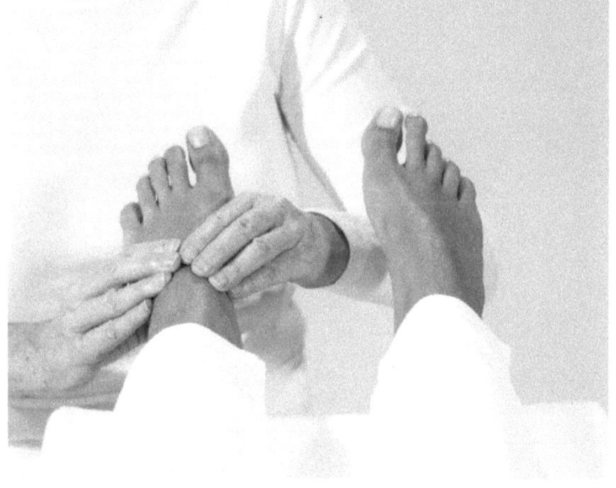

2: Around the ankle to the lower lymph reflex

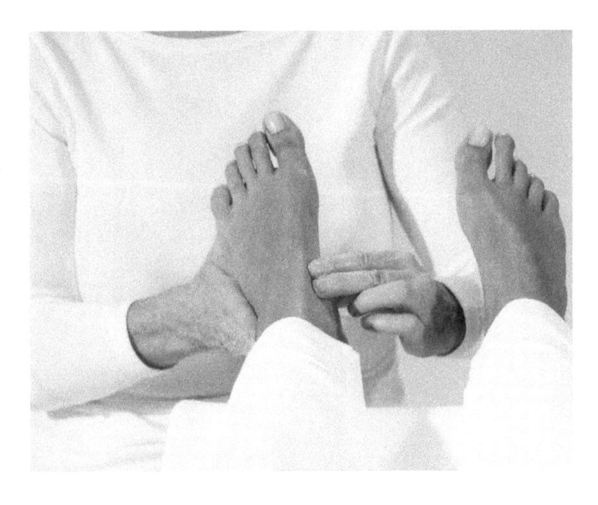

3: Support the foot with the hand on the lateral edge

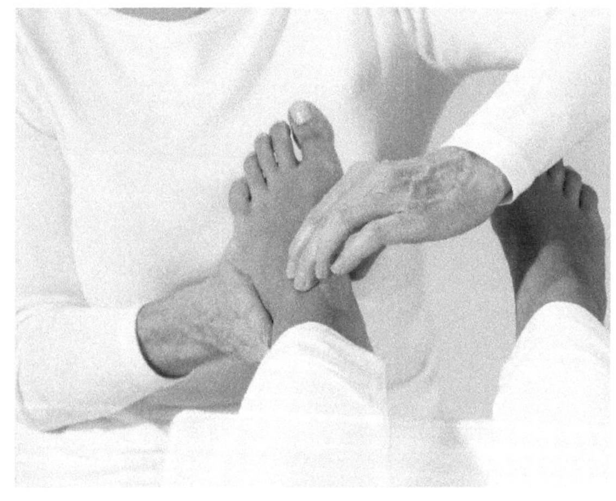

4: With the index and middle finger of the free hand hook across the lower lymph reflexes

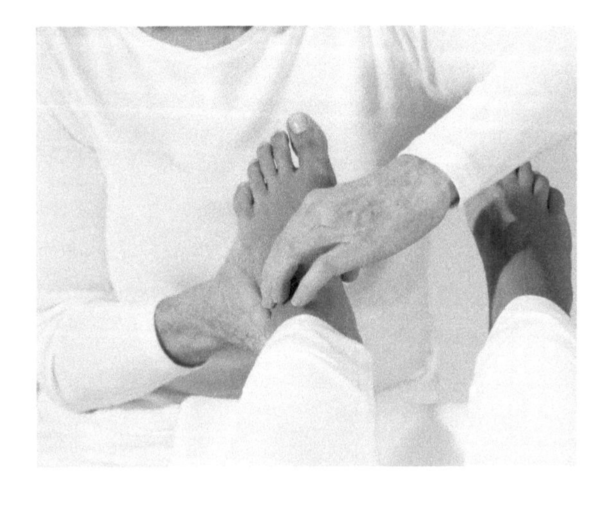

5: From medial to lateral

7b: Lower lymph (lateral to medial), cisterna chyli, thoracic duct & subclavian vein

Change hands and return from lateral to medial back across the lower lymph reflexes, towards the cisterna chyli.

As the returning hand sweeps across the lower lymph reflex, aim for the head of the navicular bone with the middle finger. Change hands and place your thumb on the head of the navicular and slide into the cisterna chyli reflex on the medial edge of the cuneiform bone, press gently and pause (as before in step 2b (i, ii, iii)). See Fig 22.

Thumb walk up the thoracic duct reflex along the medial edge of the first metatarsal.

At the base of the big toe, change from thumb to index finger and slide across the dorsal base of the big toe, and down between the first two metatarsals to the subclavian vein. Repeat 3 times.

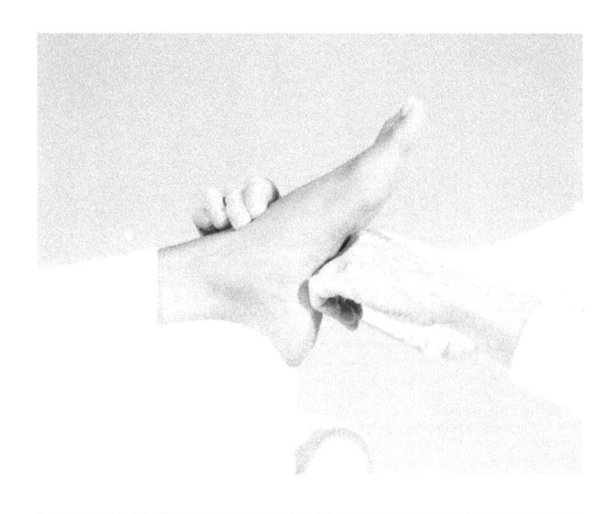

6: Change hands and return from lateral to medial back across the lower lymph reflexes

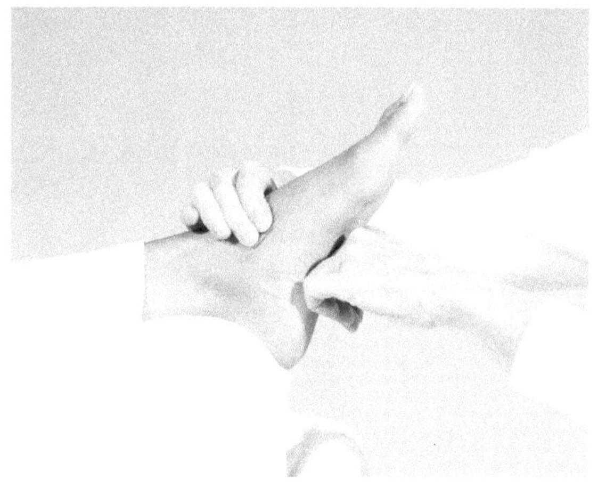

7: Towards the cisterna chyli. Aim towards the head of the navicular

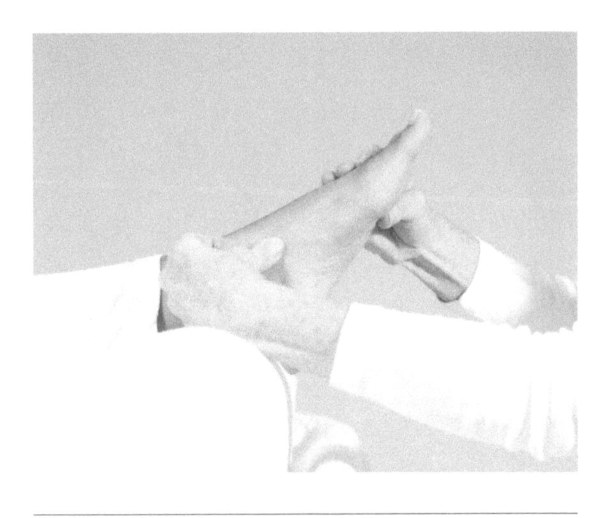

8: Change hands and place your thumb on the head of the navicular

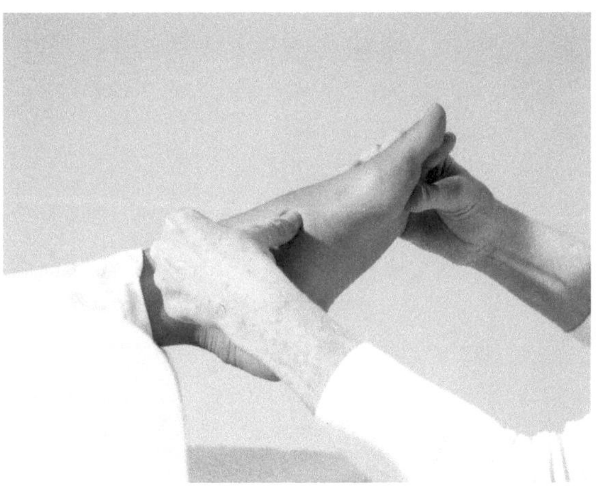

9: Slide into the cisterna chyli reflex on the medial edge of the cuneiform bone

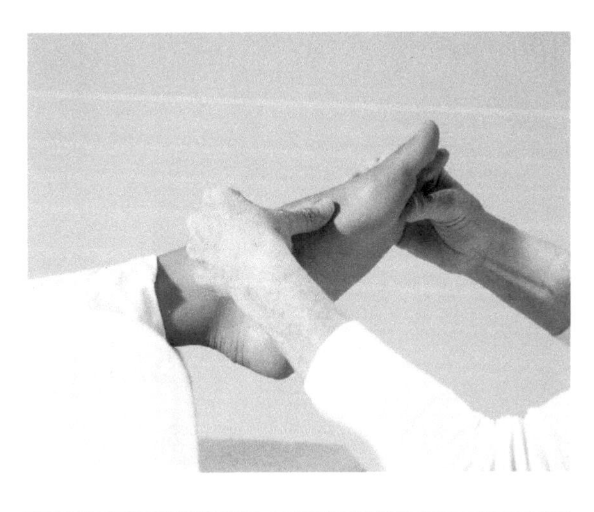

10: Thumb walk up the thoracic duct reflex along the medial edge of the first metatarsal

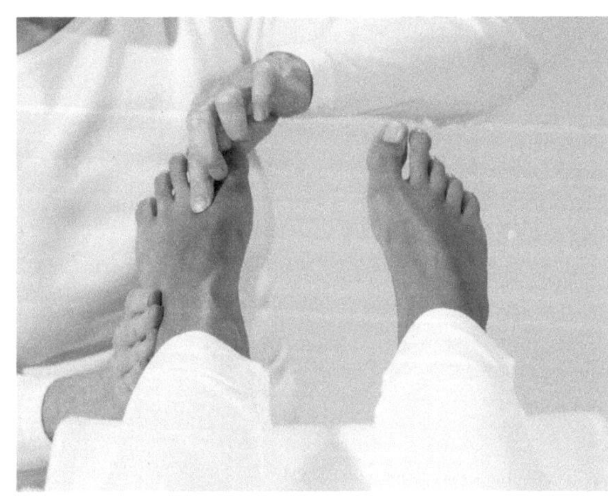

11: At the base of the big toe, change from thumb to index finger and slide across the dorsal base of the big toe, and down between the first two metatarsals to the subclavian vein

Summary of steps 7a & 7b as one move

- Light effleurage down the dorsal with both hands
- Sweep around the ankles
- Hook across the lower lymph from medial to lateral
- Return from lateral to medial
- Into the cisterna chyli
- Up the thoracic duct
- Into the subclavian vein

Repeat 3a & 3b together 3 times.

Step 8: Breast reflex

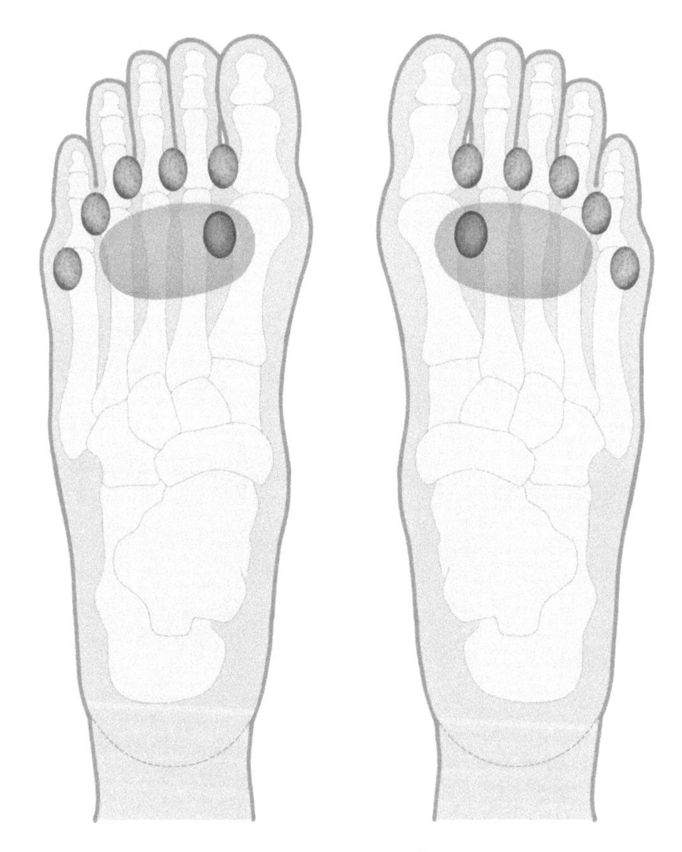

Fig. 32: **Breast reflex**

Work the dorsal breast reflex, from medial to lateral, lateral to medial, and back to the subclavian vein.

Medial to lateral - use a light pressure to work down between each of the metatarsals.

Lateral to medial - use a light circular move with the emphasis drawing up towards the upper lymph reflexes and to the subclavian vein.

Repeat 3 times.

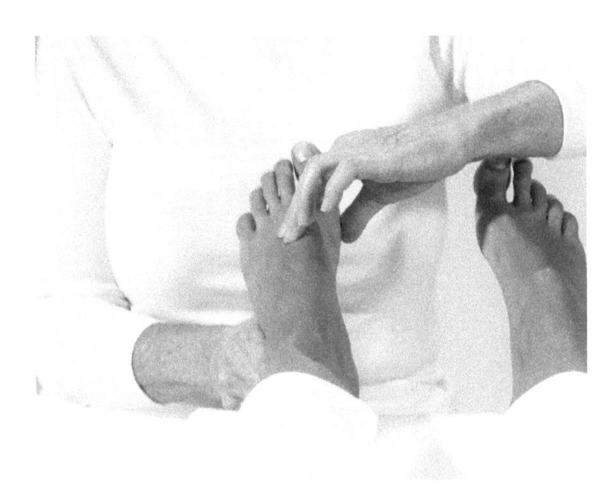

1: Work the dorsal breast reflex, from medial to lateral

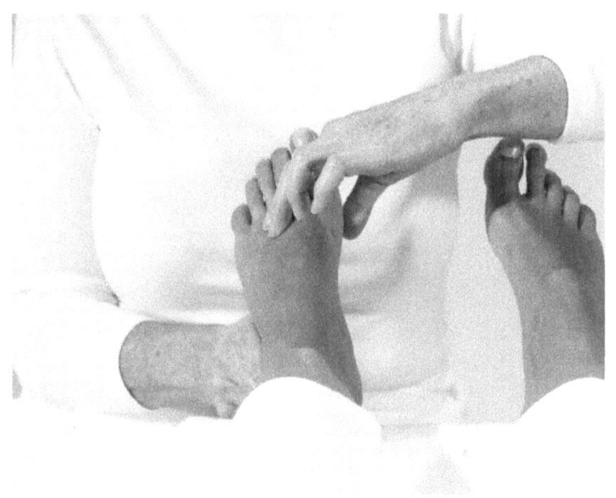

2: Use a light pressure to work down between each of the metatarsals

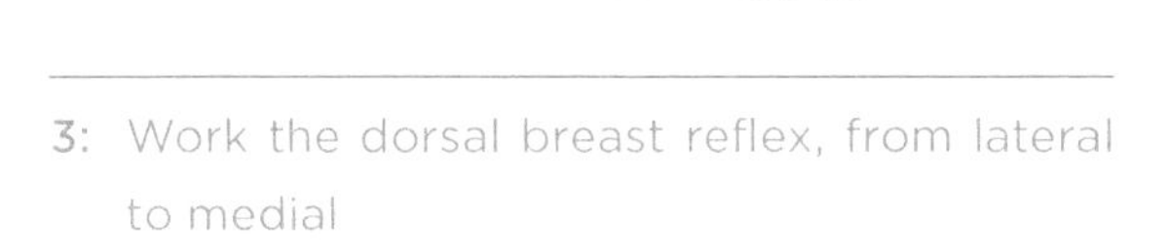

3: Work the dorsal breast reflex, from lateral to medial

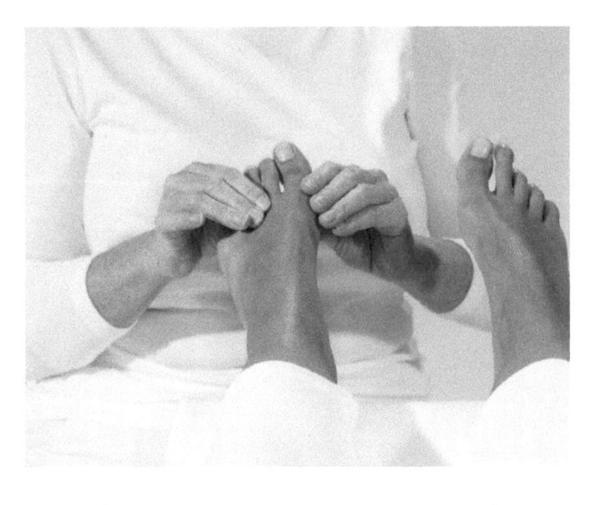

4: Use a light circular movement

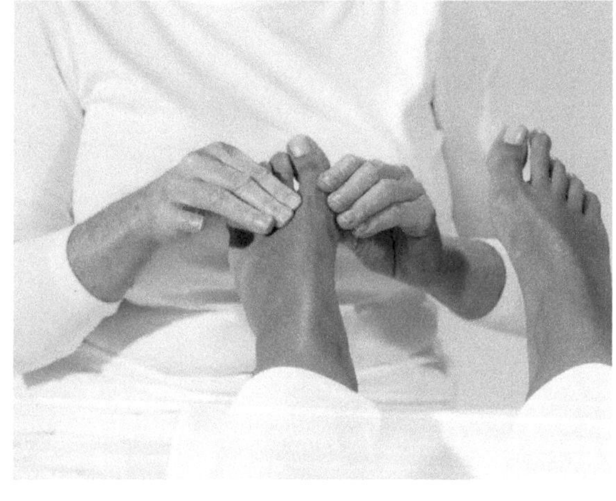

5: Emphasise drawing up towards the upper lymph reflexes

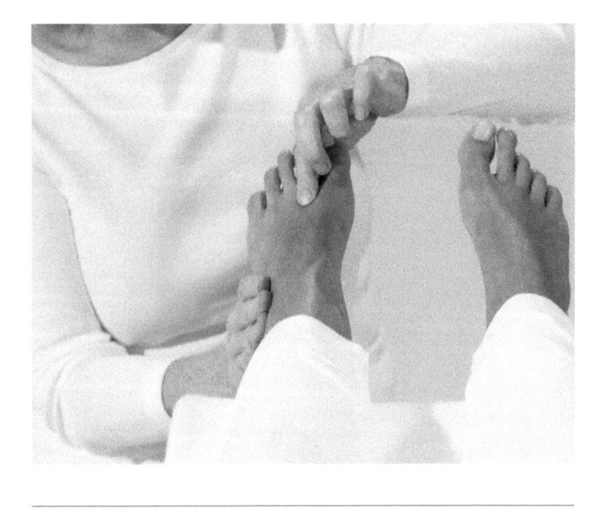

6: Into the subclavian vein

Step 9: Arm

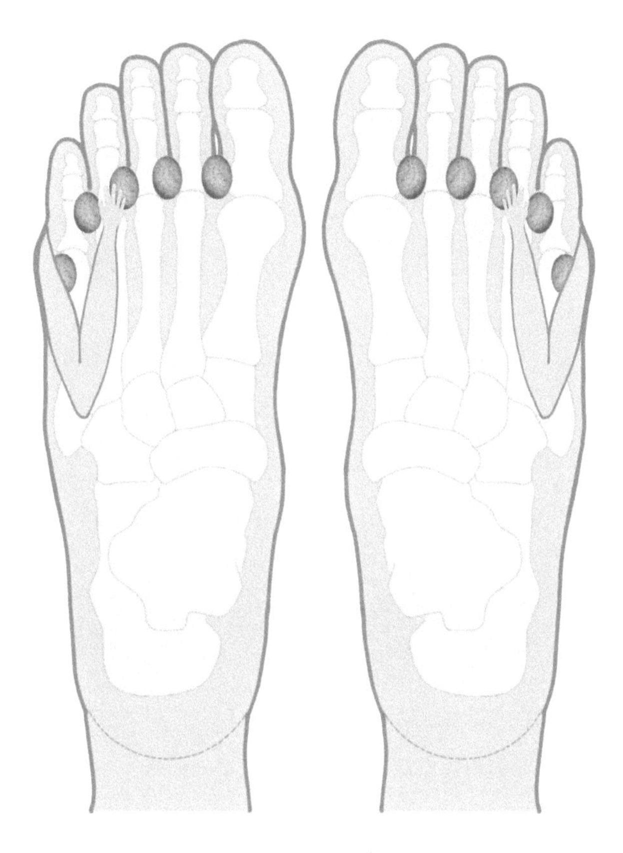

Fig. 33: **Arm reflex**

From the subclavian vein reflex, circle across the upper lymph reflexes as before (see steps 4, 5 & 6) to the deltoid at the top of the arm reflex on the lateral edge of the foot.

Work the arm from the lateral shoulder deltoid as far as the wrist and hand reflex. Thumb or finger walk down to the elbow reflex (medial proximal end of the fifth metatarsal), and from the elbow to the wrist and hand reflex just below the fourth toe (distal head of the fourth metatarsal).

Reverse this to return from the wrist and hand reflex, back to the elbow, and up to the shoulder. Circle back across the upper lymph reflexes from lateral to medial, into the subclavian vein. Repeat 3 times.

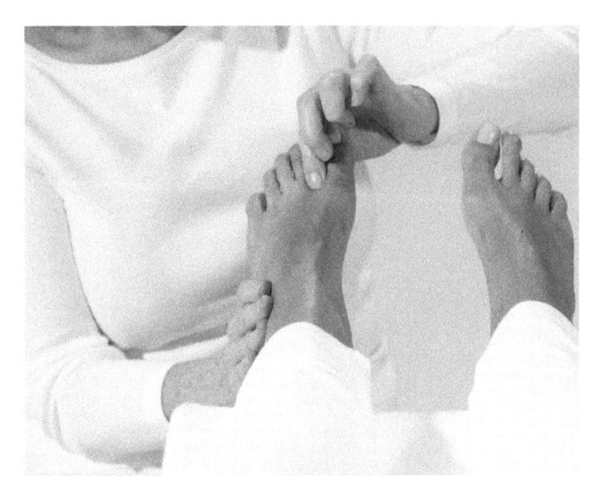

1: Slide towards the toes from the subclavian vein reflex into the first of the upper lymph reflexes

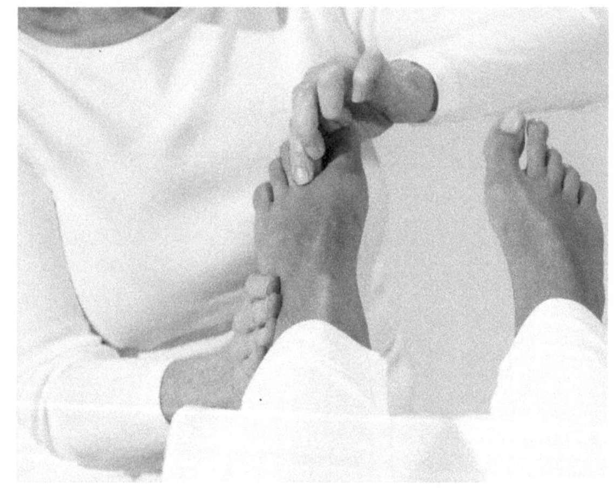

2: Work from medial to lateral, keep the working hand high and use a circular movement in each upper lymph reflex

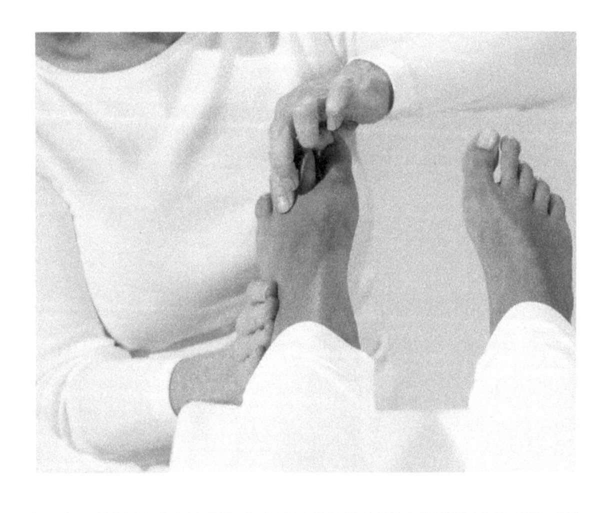

3: Transition smoothly between each of the five upper lymph reflexes

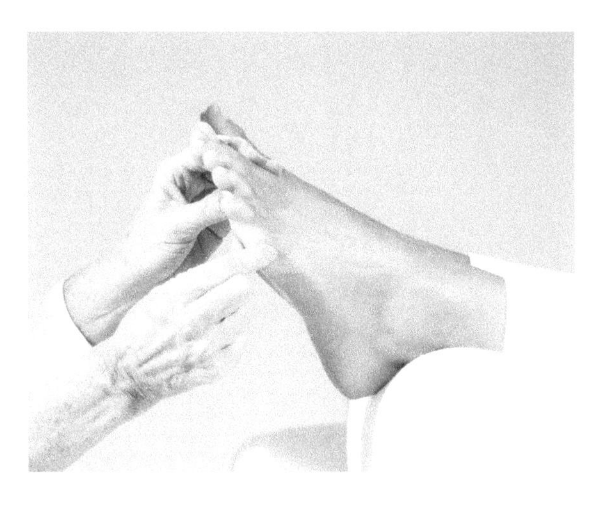

4: Thumb or finger walk the upper arm reflexes from the deltoid to the elbow

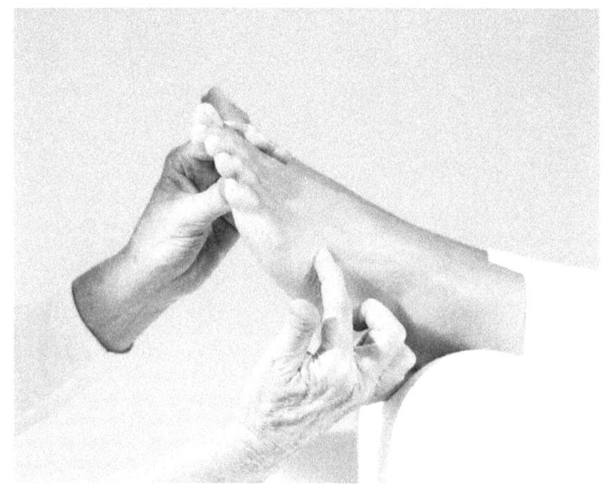

5: Elbow reflex (medial proximal end of the fifth metatarsal)

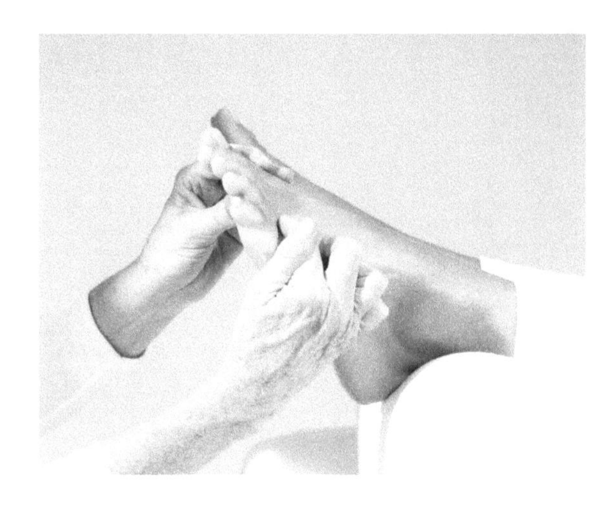

6: From the elbow to the wrist and hand reflex just below the fourth toe (distal head of the fourth metatarsal)

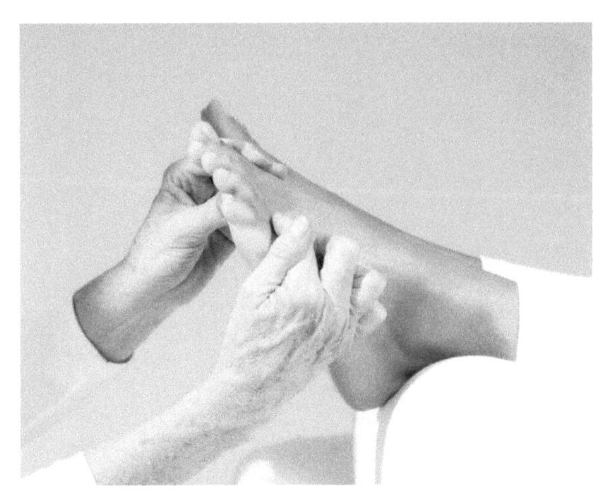

7: Reverse these steps to return from the wrist and hand reflex

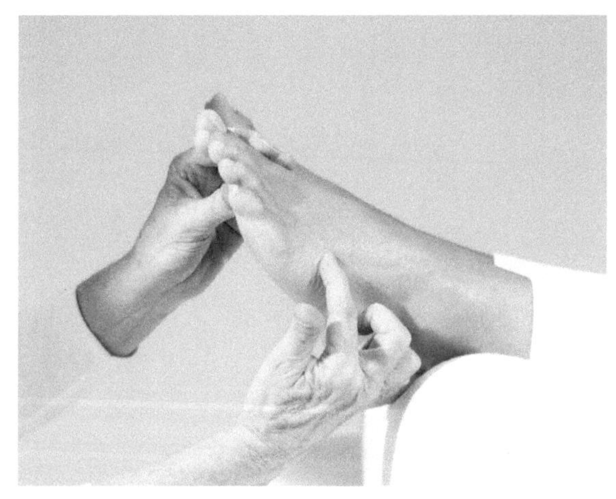

8: Back to the elbow

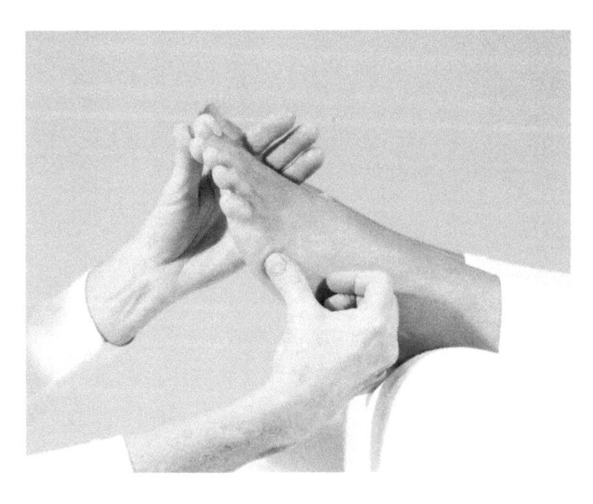

9: From the elbow up to the deltoid

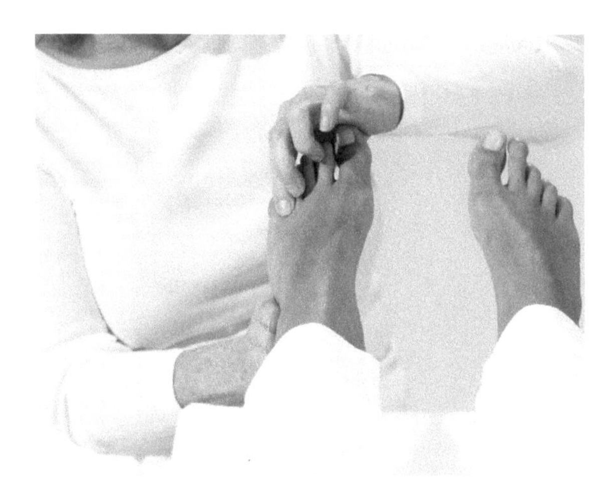

10: Keep the working hand high and work the upper lymph reflexes from above

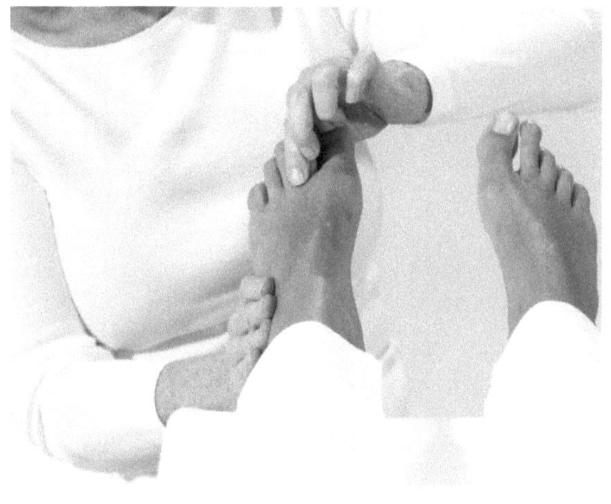

11: Use circular movements across the upper lymph reflexes from lateral to medial

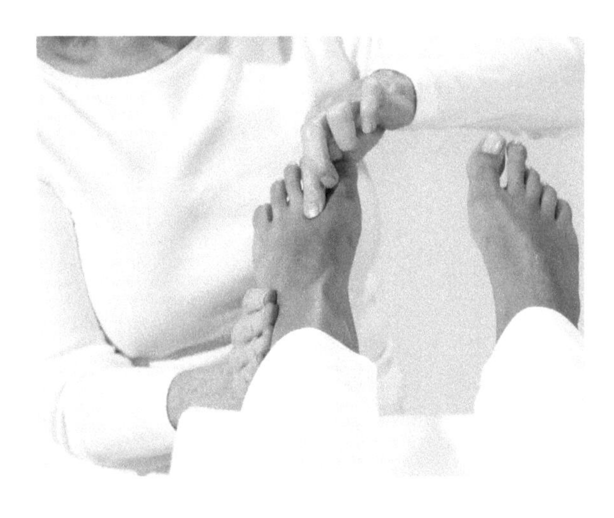

12: Keep the lymph draining back towards the subclavian vein

Step 10: Spleen reflex (left foot only)

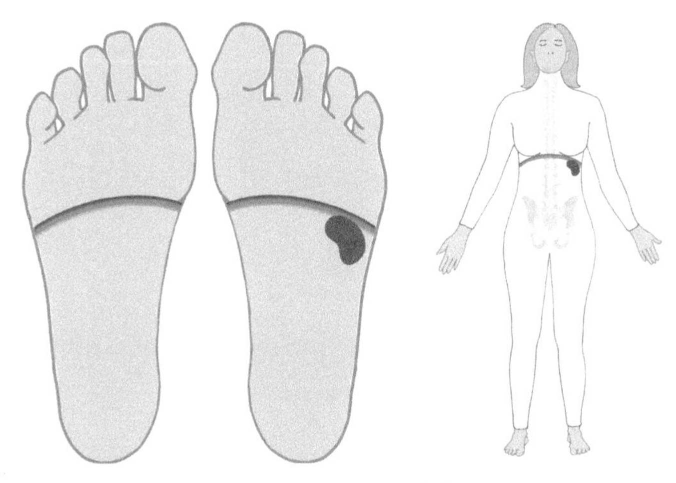

Fig. 34: **Spleen**

Work the spleen reflex with the pad of the right thumb, slowly and deliberately 5 times in a clockwise direction.

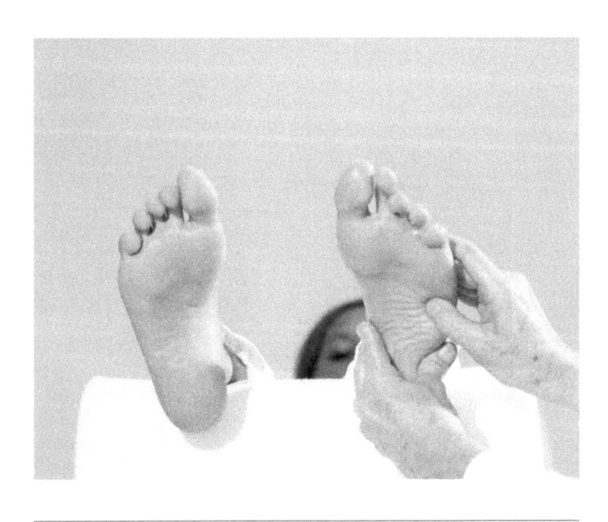

1: Work the spleen reflex 5 times in a clockwise direction

Step 11: Kidney to bladder flush

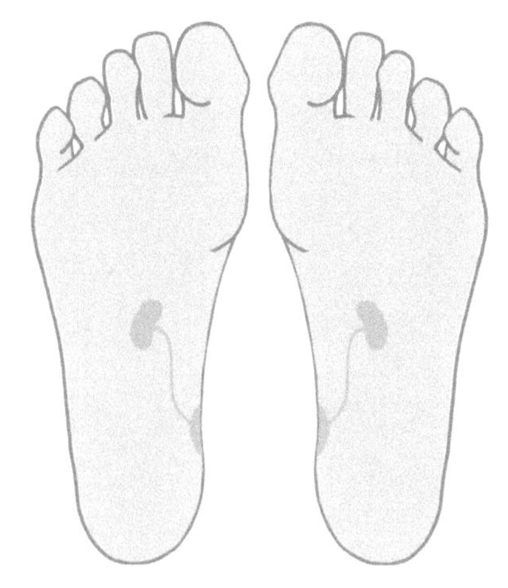

Fig. 35: Kidney to bladder reflex

Kidney to bladder flush to support the process and elimination of waste. Gently sweep from kidney to bladder reflexes 3 times.

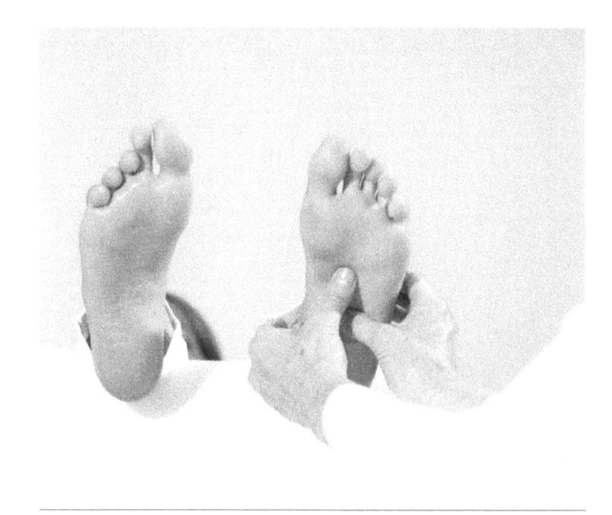

1: Kidney to bladder flush

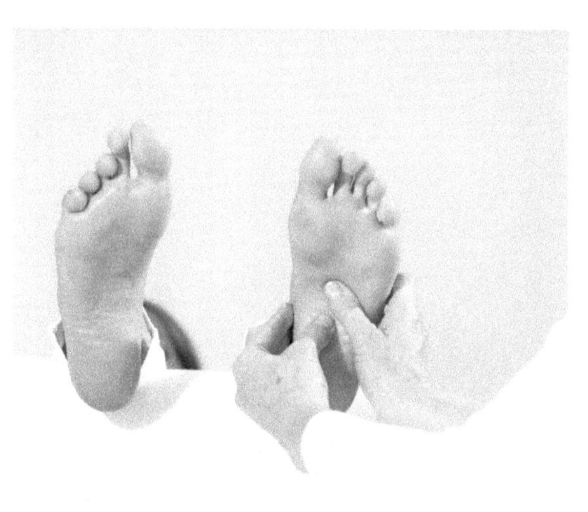

2: Gently sweep from kidney to bladder

Step 12: Linking

At the end of the treatment, after three feet have been worked, (right-left-right, or left-right-left) finish the treatment by linking the cervical lymph nodes reflex to axillary lymph nodes.

One foot at a time, continue to link until any sensations subside.

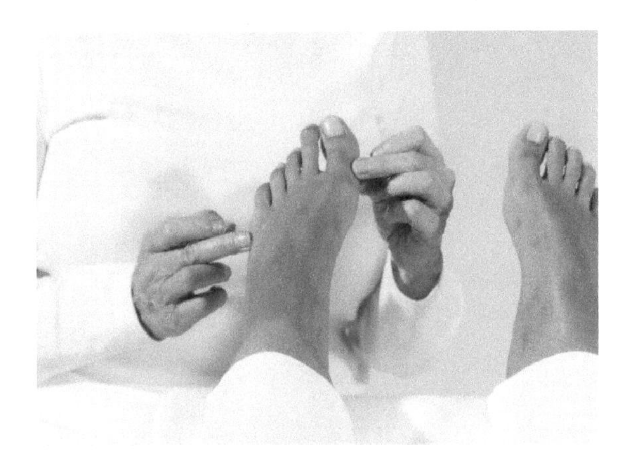

1: Link cervical lymph nodes to axilla reflexes

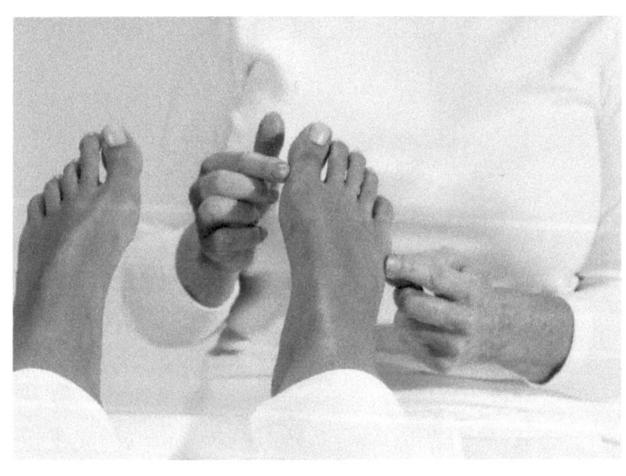

2: Repeat on the other foot

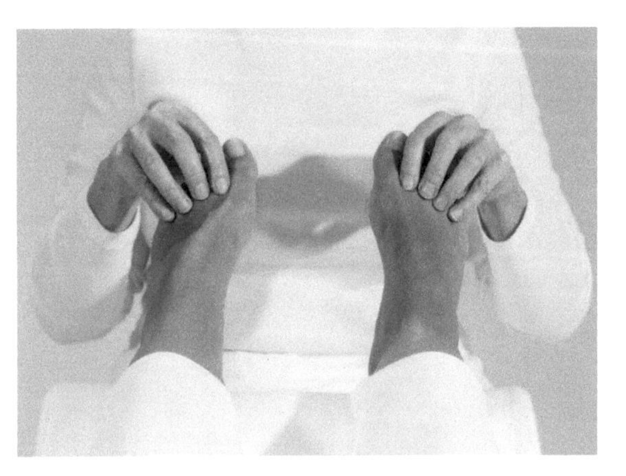

3: Finish the RLD treatment with the upper lymph hold

Finish the RLD sequence with the upper lymph hold, by gently placing the fingertips on each of the upper lymph reflexes, lightly holding both feet together.

Clients may report feeling movement or strange sensations that they often find difficult to describe. *"This might sound a bit weird, but..."*

Examples of these sensations include tingling, rippling, a flow, a trickle, light pins and needles, feathering, a wave, or a sensation in the bladder.

When linking, "less is more": less pressure usually equals more sensations. Touch the reflex with hardly any pressure and hold the position for a moment, and gradually ease away and break contact from the skin. Hold the position and ask the client if they feel "more or less", with the linking finger on or off. In response to their feedback adjust accordingly.

If the concept of linking is new to you, prepare to be surprised and delighted!

Summary of RLD for unilateral secondary lymphoedema of the arm

Start the treatment on the side that corresponds with the same side of the body as the normal arm.

Repeat on the side corresponding with the swollen arm.

Return to the normal side and repeat the sequence.

RLD can be done on feet or hands.

Summary of RLD reflexes

1. Diaphragm Repeat 5 x	• Start at the lateral edge - work the diaphragm from lateral to medial - medial to lateral • Finish at the medial edge
2. Down, up & in 2a. Spinal cord 2b. Cisterna chyli, thoracic duct, SCV Repeat 3 x	• Work down the spinal cord (C1–T12) and beyond to L3 • Swap hands and press into cisterna chyli • Work up the thoracic duct • Into the subclavian vein (SCV)
3. Opening up at the neck and clearing the back 3a. Cervical lymph nodes 3b. Upper trapezius Repeat 3 x	• Work the cervical lymph nodes • Thumb walk across the back of the neck • Circle along the upper trapezius & down around the scapula • Return from lateral to medial to the SCV
Wake up the upper lymph to make space 4. Upper lymph Repeat 3 x	• Start at the SCV • Gently slide up towards the first upper lymph reflex • Circle each reflex from medial to lateral • Work the axillary lymph nodes • Circle lateral to medial and return to the SCV
Clear the shoulder 5. Lateral shoulder Repeat 3 x	• Start at the SCV • Gently slide up towards the first upper lymph reflex • Circle each reflex from medial to lateral • Work the deltoid/lateral shoulder • Circle lateral to medial and return to the SCV
Pump under the arm 6. Axillary lymph nodes Repeat 3 x	• Start at the SCV • Gently slide up towards the first upper lymph reflex • Circle each reflex from medial to lateral • Pump the axillary lymph nodes reflex • Circle lateral to medial and return to the SCV

Clear the lower lymph 7. Lower lymph Repeat 3 x	• With both hands sweep down over the dorsal • Hook across the lower lymph from medial to lateral • Return lateral to medial across the lower lymph towards the cisterna chyli • Work up the thoracic duct into the SCV
Clear the breast 8. Breast Repeat 3 x	• Work the breast from medial to lateral • Return from lateral to medial with emphasis up towards the upper lymph reflexes into the SCV
Clear the arm 9. Arm Repeat 3 x	• Start at the SCV • Gently slide up towards the first upper lymph reflex • Circle each reflex from medial to lateral • At the deltoid work the arm to the wrist & hand • Circle lateral to medial and return to the SCV
Support elimination 10. Spleen Repeat 5 x	• Left side only - work the spleen in a clockwise direction
11. Kidneys and bladder Repeat 3 x	• Left & right - gentle kidney to bladder flush
Linking to finish 12. Linking	• Link cervical lymph nodes and axilla • Light touch hold to upper lymph reflexes

NOTE: During treatment patients may report feeling movement, rippling, a wave, air, feathering, heaviness, or sensation in the bladder. Continue to hold the light touch linking until the sensation subsides.

RLD hand reflexes

There are times when it is not possible to work on the feet, or you may like to give yourself some RLD.

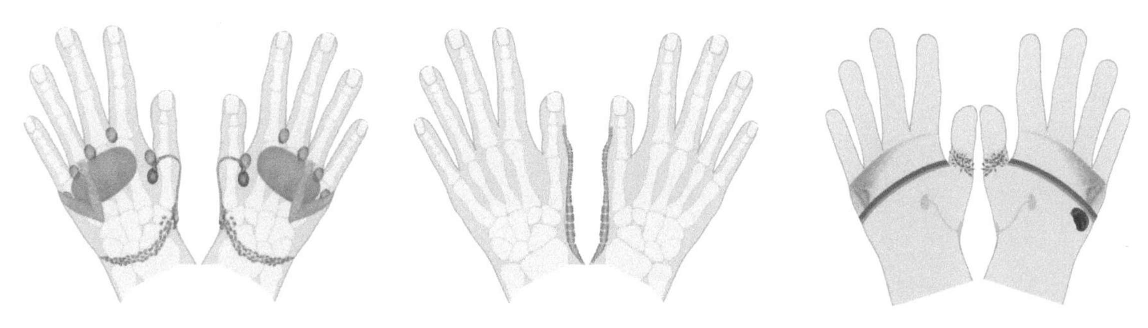

Fig. 36: **Hand reflexes for RLD**

Home help tip

Sometimes a client will ask if there is anything they can do between appointments. I recommend 3 of each of steps 4, 5 & 6 on the hands. Work 3 hands. Begin on the good side, then do it on the swollen side and repeat on the good side to finish. This can be done daily.

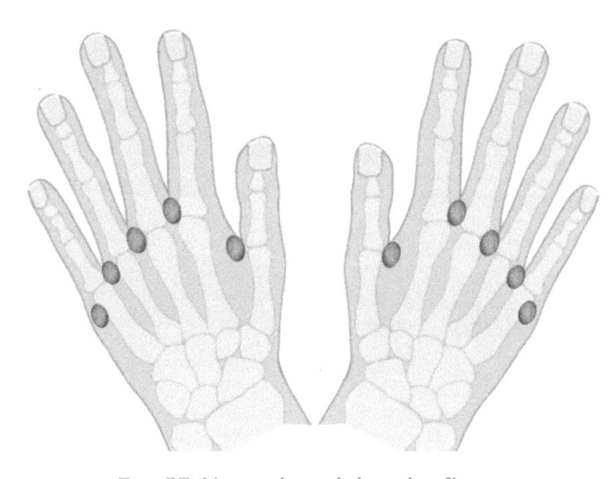

Fig. 37: **Upper lymph hand reflexes**

Integrating RLD

Since first developing RLD, it has become obvious that the protocol has quite a profoundly positive effect on clients with many other non-cancer related, inflammatory and auto-immune conditions, not just lymphoedema of the arm. Simple adjustments can also be made to use RLD for clients with lymphoedema swelling in other areas.

There is a growing body of anecdotal evidence to support this through clinical experience with clients, RLD case studies (see Chapter 10 on page 186) and treatments that are received during the practical sessions on RLD courses. These continue to delight and amaze everybody present who either feel it first-hand or see the benefits in others, and we can all learn so much from this.

Sometimes the physical movement of lymph can trigger a kind of psychological peristalsis of stagnant emotions. When this happens, people may experience quite a significant emotional release. After letting go they feel physically and psychologically lighter. There is a wonderful sense of renewal, clarity and homeostasis.

The following information explains how to adapt the treatment when clients present with other problems now that you understand the first principles of the original RLD protocol. It can be used as an effective stand-alone treatment, and ultimately provides a set of tools for the reflexology tool box, one that is easy to integrate into your everyday practice.

When treatment planning, remember with lymphoedema swelling the aim is to create a space in the nearest functioning area of lymph nodes to cause an effect on the drainage function.

Understand the pathology of the presenting condition, where the blockage is or the cause of the swelling - this will help you to safely adapt any reflexology treatment to best suit the individual along with other influencing factors, symptoms and side effects and interactions with medication. Everyone is different, so always make an informed choice.

RLD & lymphoedema swelling of the legs

In cases of lymphoedema of the leg or legs, follow steps 1-7 of the protocol to get things moving. Next, instead of steps 8 & 9, the breast and arm, sweep back down to the lower lymph reflexes (7a). Work from medial to lateral all the way around to the top of the leg reflex (hip reflex), a small dent in the calcaneus bone. Work the reflexes of the leg from hip to knee and from knee to foot with a thumb or finger walk. Reverse this move and follow the same reflexes back from foot to knee, knee to hip (dent in calcaneus). Sweep back across the lower lymph as with step 7b. Aim for the head of the navicular with the middle finger, then swap hands and use the thumb to slide into the cisterna chyli reflex on the medial edge of the cuneiform bone. Pause for a moment before thumb walking up the thoracic duct reflex and into the subclavian vein. Repeat this move a few times. You could also include some ankle rocking and dorsiflex pumping.

RLD & bilateral secondary lymphoedema of the arms

In the case of a client with a double mastectomy, lymphoedema can develop in both arms. RLD can be adapted to help these clients.

Work steps 1-7 as before to get things moving and create a space. The breast and arm reflexes steps 8 & 9 are worked slightly differently. Medial to lateral breast reflex is as before, down between the metatarsals, but a different pathway is taken back to the subclavian vein. Instead of circling across the breast reflex from lateral to medial, sweep down the dorsal and work as for 7a & 7b. The aim is to take the lymph to the nearest functioning group of lymph nodes: in this case via the lower lymph, effectively taking a diversion, the long way round back to the subclavian vein. Same for the arm: circle from medial to lateral across the upper lymph reflexes to the arm reflex and work as before to the wrist and hand reflex. The return route is slightly different. Work the arm reflex from hand and wrist to elbow and up towards the shoulder as far as the armpit (under the distal head of the fifth metatarsal), stop and sweep down the dorsal as steps 7a & 7b, and bring it back up the thoracic duct reflex to the subclavian vein as before.

RLD & primary lymphoedema and lipoedema

For clients with primary lymphoedema and/or lipoedema it is a good idea to use the full protocol, and include the reflexes for the arms and legs in the sequence.

RLD & inflammatory and auto-immune conditions

It makes sense that if RLD can cause an effect on the drainage function of the lymphatic system, indicated in the results of the research (see Chapter 9 on page 167), it has the potential to also affect the immune system. This might account for why RLD appears to help so many clients with inflammatory, auto-immune conditions.

When working with this client group (people with inflammatory, auto-immune disorders), include RLD as part of the reflexology - just work 2 feet. This can be given as a short stand-alone treatment or easily integrated as part of a longer reflexology session depending on the client.

The use of RLD as a short treatment (2 feet only) for clients with fibromyalgia and chronic fatigue syndrome is less likely to trigger the same healing crisis as with a standard reflexology session for these clients. The fluent gentle nature of this treatment is ideal for this client group.

Clients with any of these conditions often feel bruised in the subclavian vein and cisterna chyli reflexes. This is a recurring theme in all cases where inflammation is involved, or if the lymphatic system is somehow compromised with an auto-immune condition or clients with a stubborn virus or common cold that's hard to shift. These two reflexes are very useful for the reflexology tool box, as they will highlight imbalances in the system.

As previously mentioned, I prefer to avoid the power of suggestion when it comes to explaining what people might feel. For me less is more. Even when someone says, "I can feel a sort of tingling, is that normal?" I avoid the question with a vague response of, "Everybody's different, let's wait and see how you feel at the end." Silence is a skill and by holding the space without trying to fill it, the client is more likely to find their own words to describe what they can feel.

The flip side of this is saying too much, then if the client doesn't notice anything, they might assume that it is not working. However, if measurements have been taken, the undeniable evidence is right there!

Now that you understand how to implement RLD the next chapter is about making an informed choice with the individual cautions and contra-indications for best practice.

Reflection

- RLD applies the principle of MLD to the reflexes of the feet and hands
- The aim of RLD is to invoke the natural drainage function of the body
- The original protocol is for unilateral lymphoedema of the arm
- RLD can be used as a stand-alone treatment or adapted accordingly for clients with other presenting conditions

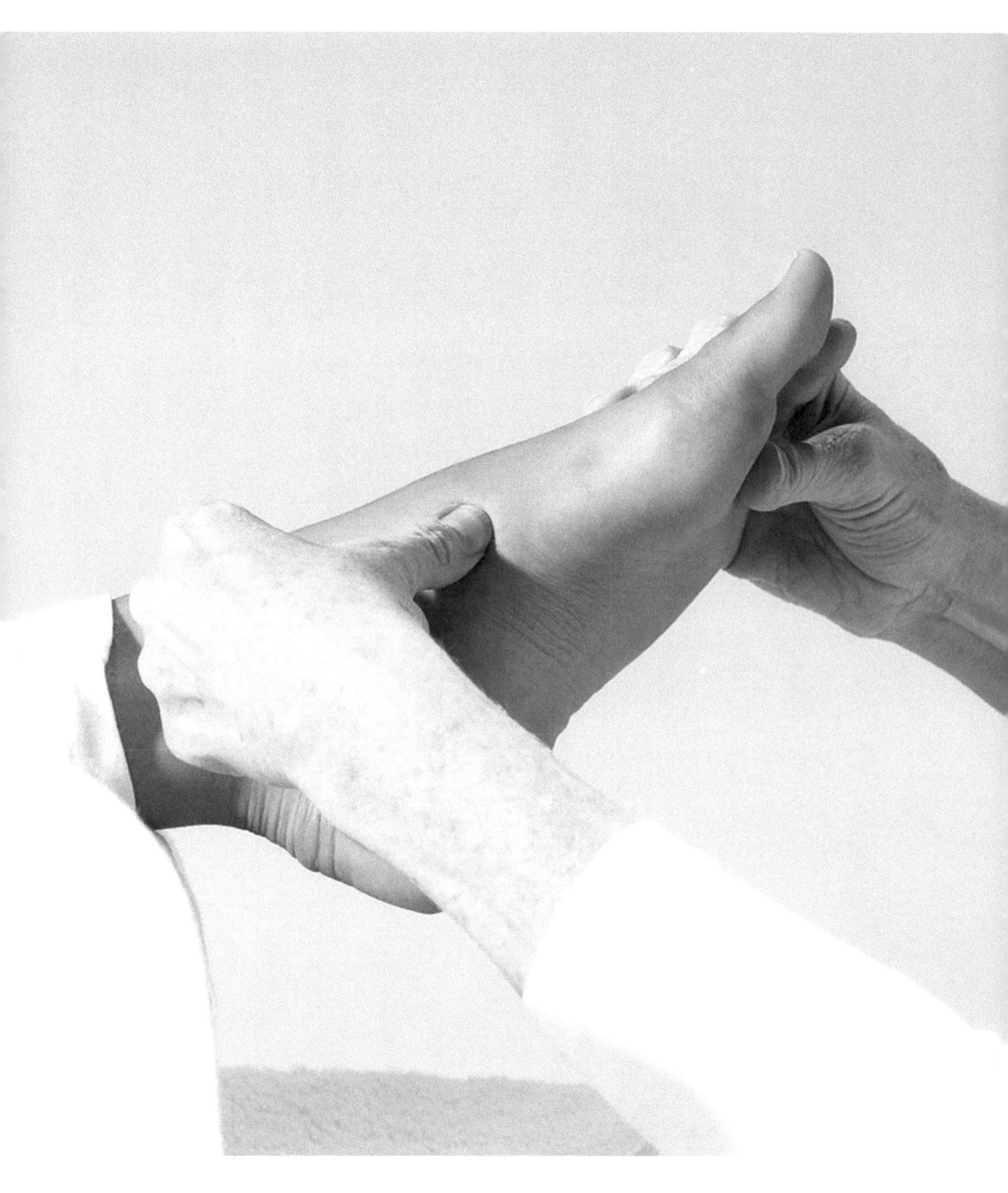

Chapter 7
Clinical Reasoning and Best Practice

Expectation

This chapter is a discussion about safe practice, cautions and contra-indications for RLD and the importance of making an informed therapeutic choice during treatment planning. It is the responsibility of each reflexology practitioner to adapt treatment accordingly to best suit the recipient.

Throughout this book I have repeatedly mentioned the importance of understanding the pathology of presenting conditions, symptoms, side effects and medical intervention in order to deliver a safe and adapted reflexology treatment. I believe that this critical thinking approach to reflexology is the art of learning.

"Learn to question things rather than to just ask questions." - Sally Kay

In the years of working at the hospice I used to go home after the clinics and read about the symptoms of disease and the side effects of treatments and medication. This is still part of my clinical practice and it provides a certain level of understanding. These days it's so easy to ask questions on social media, but this actually deprives us of essential knowledge and the ability to apply our own clinical reasoning.

Reflexology client groups are all different and each has its own unique set of guidelines. As a reflexology practitioner, work within your limits of competence and training.

In my experience, knowledge, training and peer support helped to give me the confidence as a reflexology practitioner and to develop the ability to adapt and treat clients with complex and life limiting conditions. Ironically this client group may be excluded sometimes from having reflexology due to fear and lack of understanding with "text book" contra-indications and cautions, yet they might be the people who benefit the most from receiving the caring touch of a reflexologist.

I have worked as a complementary therapist, primarily using reflexology, with patients at all stages of their cancer journey, and other life limiting conditions, from diagnosis, through treatments and surgery. Often I have heard survivors talk about how anxious they felt when the hospital discharged them after successfully treating the disease.

"Good news, we'll see you again in 12 months for a check-up."

This can be an extremely stressful time of mixed emotions for many people. They may worry about the uncertainty of the future, some feel fear or guilt and have lost their confidence. Reflexology in its many guises can provide a wonderful support as people come to terms with what they've been through and learn to how manage a whole new set of health related worries or anxiety which can easily escalate.

Reflexology in the palliative care setting is different again. My experience of this includes working in both hospitals and with domiciliary visits. Two very different environments, and both have a separate set of challenges. In the hospital, access to the feet may be difficult, and so a very gentle hand reflexology might be the best option. Similarly with home visits, access to the patient can be awkward and family members may be with them, and the distress is apparent even though they put on a brave face.

In Case study 2 (Chapter 10 on page 192), the daughter wept silently as the reflexologist worked on her mother.

As she spoke her daughter wiped away a tear. She also looked exhausted and helpless, desperate for anything to relieve her mother's agony.

The ripple effect of a calming, gentle treatment is comforting to everyone present, not just the patient. Reflexology is a gift to all under these circumstances.

I had the privilege of treating this lady on two further occasions before she passed away. Her daughter was grateful that her mother had been helped in such a positive way.

I have also worked on chemotherapy wards, giving a gentle, relaxing reflexology treatment to help patients with anxiety or a needle phobia, although definitely not RLD at this time. As previously mentioned, the cytotoxic chemotherapy drugs have a job to do.

Reflexology comes in many different applications and modalities, and all of these techniques are subject to interpretation by the practitioner. This makes it difficult to follow hard and fast rules, and when it comes to treatment planning, because one size does not fit all!

Therefore, and to ensure safe practice, it is always important to understand how the presenting conditions of the client can affect the body, and the impact disease has, physically and psychologically, on anyone who comes for reflexology.

Consider the diagnosis, the pathology of the disease and the symptoms of the condition as well as the side effects and interactions of any medication or other intervention. This must be understood when making an informed choice on how best to adapt and implement a reflexology treatment.

Reflexologists who work with patients and clients who have been diagnosed and treated for cancer may have undertaken further training. Remember that each person is different and their wellbeing will depend on many factors. This includes the initial diagnosis, the prognosis, the stage of the disease, different treatments and the side effects and symptoms of all of this. In some cases patients present with other complex medical health problems, plus high levels of anxiety and emotional distress.

All that said, to ensure safe practice the following contra-indications need to be considered before using the original RLD protocol for clients with breast cancer related lymphoedema. These must be observed together with all other cautions in relation to reflexology treatment.

Contra-indications for RLD

These conditions are contra-indicated in RLD:

- Deep vein thrombosis (DVT)
- Pulmonary embolism
- Cellulitis
- Undiagnosed swelling
- Unstable heart conditions
- Oedema due to end of life organ failure

While it's good practice to err on the side of caution, consider the risk of being too cautious. This could cause added distress for someone if you refuse them a reflexology treatment.

There are times when RLD or a full reflexology treatment may not be appropriate due to the complexities of the disease. In this case a comforting touch, even if it is just a gentle hold of the hands or feet, will be well received. I believe you can always offer something, even if it's a very light air reflexology.

Reflection

- Best practice is all about making an informed choice
- Treatment rationale is based on the presenting conditions of the individual
- Work within your limits of competence and training

Disclaimer

Reflexology practice is constantly evolving in response to the needs of those who seek the therapy. It is the responsibility of the reflexologist to maintain professional development and to work within the context of the individual policies and professional guidelines for best practice. The author, other contributors and the publisher are not responsible for any harm or damage to a person, no matter how caused, as a result of information shared in this book.

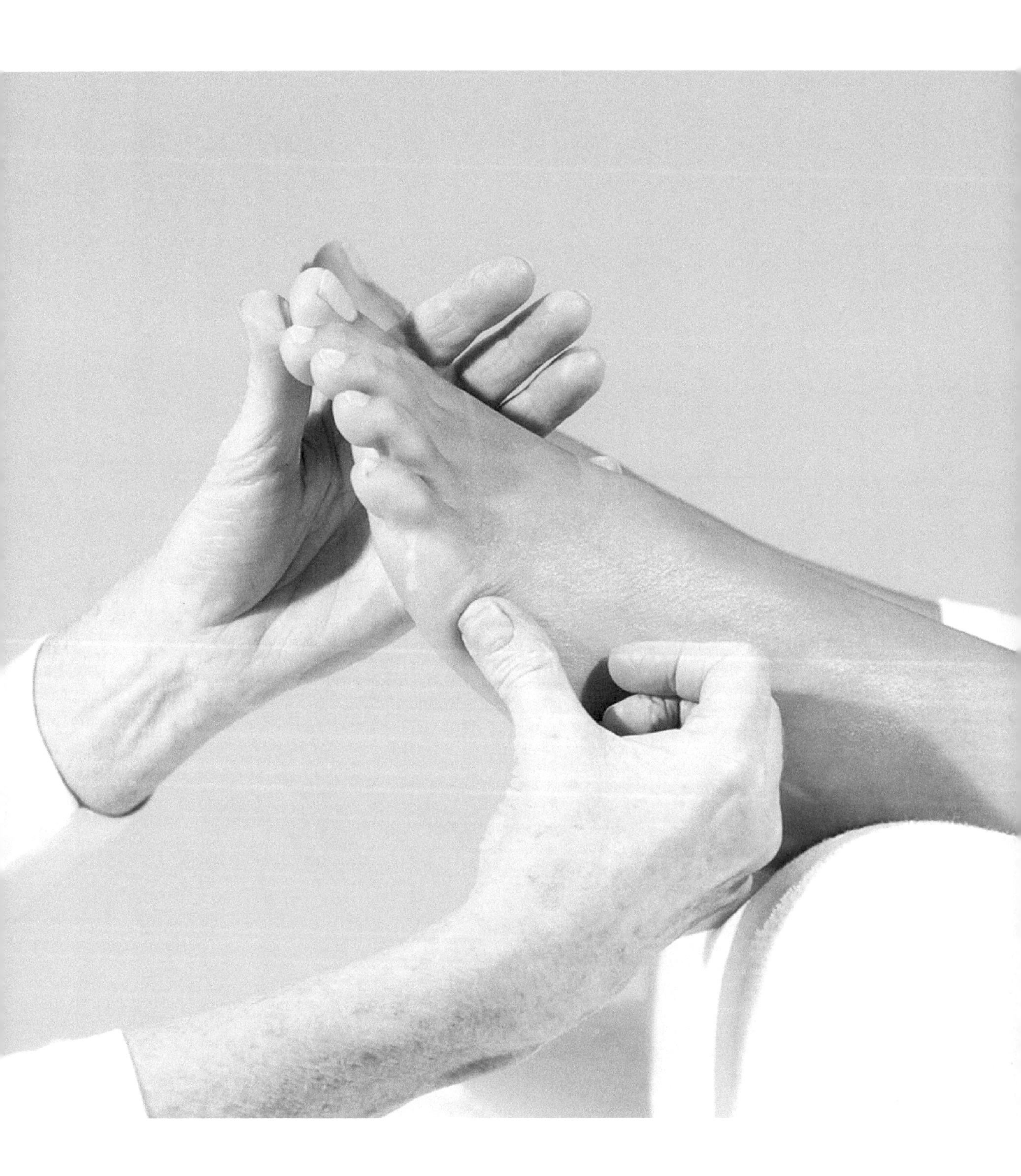

Section 4

SPEAKING VOLUMES

Chapter 8
Limb Volume Circumference Measurements

Expectation

In this chapter you will learn how to measure and calculate the volume of the arm and understand why data collection is an extremely useful skill, although not essential to the treatment. I realise that measuring and maths can be challenging (it is for me) and despite this I encourage you to follow the instructions in this chapter. Ignore the little voice inside, telling you maths is not your thing, and try it!

Using RLD to help people is the most important thing but in the words of Dr Sylvia Hood Washington:

"It is changing all the lives I am touching. Please encourage the other practitioners to document their findings for the patients. It is psychologically powerful and it encourages them to come back for the needed treatment!! Once they feel and then see in numbers the loss of fluid, they want me to do this in every session. Great tool!"

It is a worthwhile exercise to measure the circumference of the arm before and after RLD even if this is all you do. Clients with lymphoedema like to see the magic. Follow the step by step guide and prepare to be amazed! You can do it and here's how.

First let me tell you about the tape measure. The magic moment, the first time I saw RLD cause a measurable difference to the circumference of the arm.

It was a Thursday clinic in Ebbw Vale. In the weeks and months leading up to this day I had been playing with the idea of applying the principles of MLD to the lymph reflexes of the feet to try and help the patients with lymphoedema. With their full consent, I worked with them and they were more than happy to let me try. The MLD therapist had been off work with a hand injury for a long time and nothing else was available to them.

Paying careful attention to patient feedback, it seemed to be working. They all said they felt some of the same sensations during the RLD that they felt with MLD (tingling, a ripple, fluttering, almost pins and needles etc. See Chapter 6 on page 90). Clothes and jewellery appeared to be looser and there were other similarities such as the urgent need to "go", or an increase in the volume of urine immediately after RLD. I learnt a lot from their verbal and non-verbal feedback, observing similar reactions at different stages of the RLD protocol, and without the power of suggestion, it really did seem to be working!

Years of studying, first with Ted, and then for the degree, had taught me to question things. I guess I was naturally quite sceptical. Could this a placebo? Was it wishful thinking? Maybe they were just being nice; who knew?

On this particular Thursday one of the patients offered me a tape measure. I took a couple of measurements around the circumference of the proximal section of the arm, where I could see the swelling before, and then re-measured after RLD. There it was and there was no denying it, it was approximately 1.5cm smaller. I accept this was not a particularly accurate way to measure, but nevertheless it was a very exciting moment for me and everyone in the clinic that day!

The rest is history. Here was something measurable and I was going to explore the possibilities of this further. Subsequently the hospice arranged for me to visit a lymphoedema clinic in Taunton to learn how to measure accurately.

The following instructions for Limb Volume Circumference Measurements (LVCM) are what I learnt that day, taught to me by a specialist lymphoedema therapist in 2010. This method has been used in all RLD research to date.

How to measure the arm

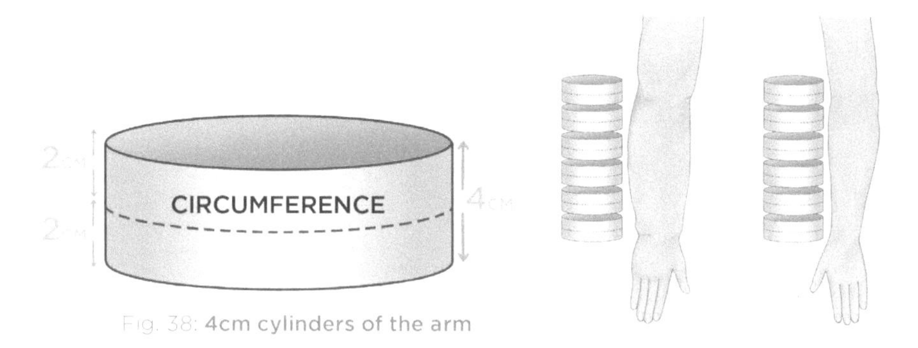

Fig. 38: 4cm cylinders of the arm

Each arm is treated like a cylinder. It is divided into a series of smaller cylinders that are 4cm in height.

The volume of each 4cm cylinder is calculated separately and then added together. The sum of this shows the volume of each arm and these figures are used to compare difference between the arms and the changes in the volume.

These figures are used to demonstrate the following:

- Volume of the whole cylinder of the arm
- Changes in distal volume
- Changes in proximal volume
- Changes in the proximal and distal ratio of swelling
- Changes to each 4cm segment

Volume is calculated from the measurements taken before and after each treatment and compared to show the changes that happen during RLD.

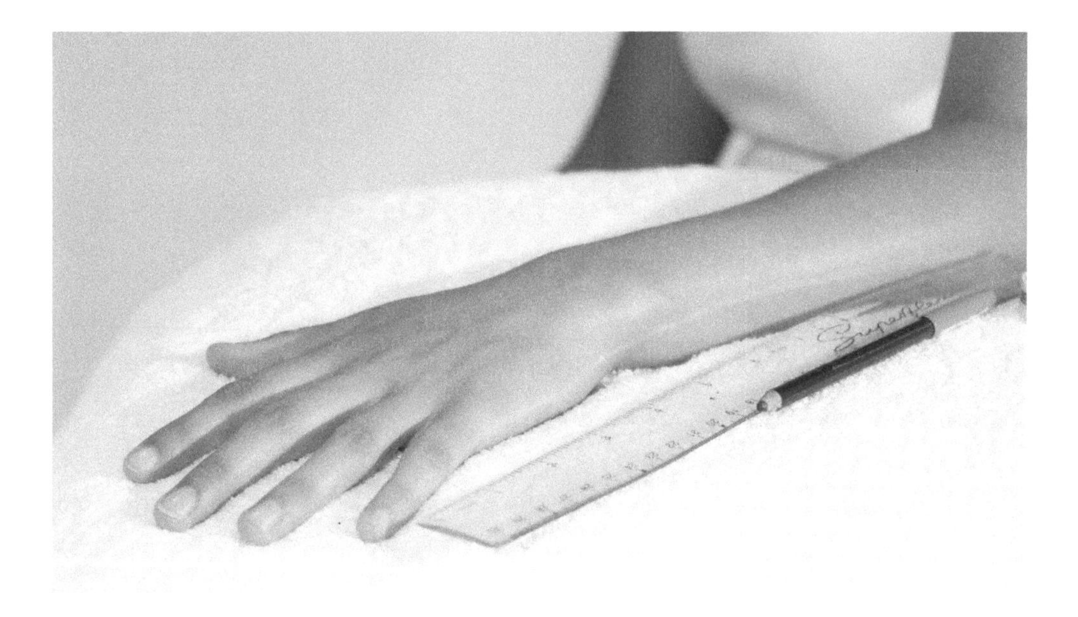

Use the following items to measure with:

- Clear plastic flexible ruler - For accuracy, mark the ruler at 4cm intervals
- Plastic coated tape measure with a loop at the end, or tension tape measure
- Skin pencil or pen for marking the skin (eye/brow liner pencil)
- Lymphoedema measurement sheet to record (see Chapter 10, Gail case study)
- Red and blue pens - This helped me to avoid confusion with left and right. I use a red pen for the swollen arm and blue/black for the normal arm.

Step by step guide to accurate measurement

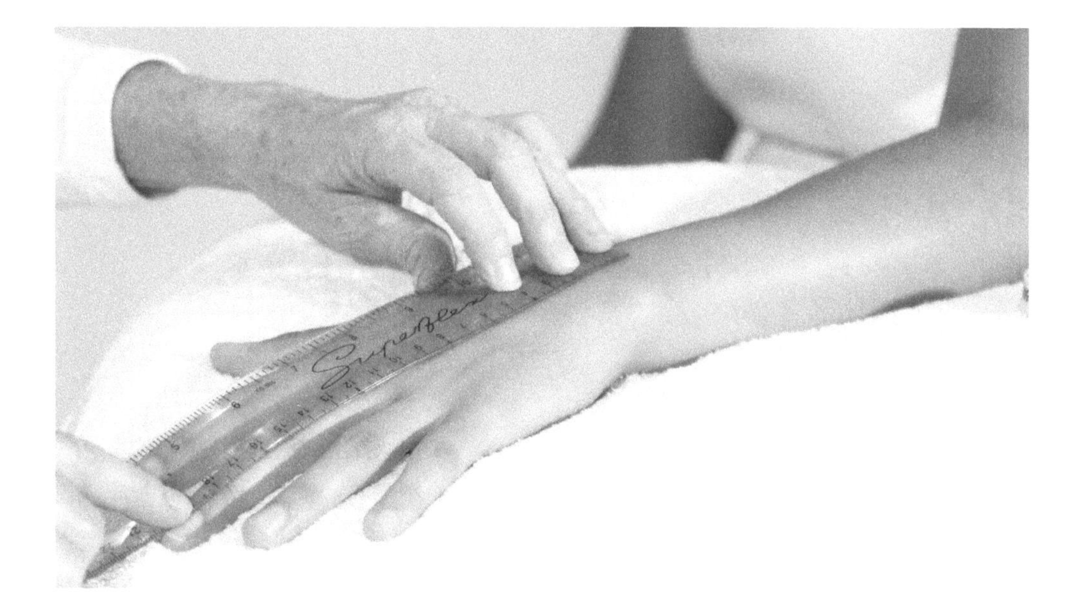

1. Sit the client in a chair with the arm extended horizontally and supported. This can be on the table or massage couch and if necessary support the arm with a cushion or pillow. Use the same set-up each time you measure the arm for consistency and like-for-like comparison.

2. Use the flexible ruler to measure along the lateral aspect of the arm from the nail bed of the middle finger to 2cm above the wrist joint.

3. Mark the first point (2cm above the wrist) and record the distance from base of middle finger nailbed. This is the fixed starting point. Use the same fixed starting point for the left and right arms and for each subsequent measurement.

4. Use the flexible ruler, pre-marked at 4cm intervals, and mark along the top of the arm at 4cm intervals as far as the axilla. Keep the line as straight as possible.

5. Use a plastic coated or tension tape measure to measure the circumference of the arm to the nearest millimetre at each marked point.

6. Record each of the circumference measurements, and as I said I find it clearer to record the swollen arm in red and normal arm in blue.

Important tips for accurate measurements

- Measure the arm in the same position every time
- Keep the arm as straight as possible
- Make sure the arm is relaxed
- Always start with the same fixed point
- Be consistent with the tension of the tape measure
- Ensure the tape measure is straight and lies smoothly around the arm
- Use the same number of measurements
- Do not include the circumference of the hand in calculations of limb volume

To see a short video "How to measure the arm RLD" subscribe to the Sally Kay YouTube channel (https://youtu.be/4rTXbZvEWz8).

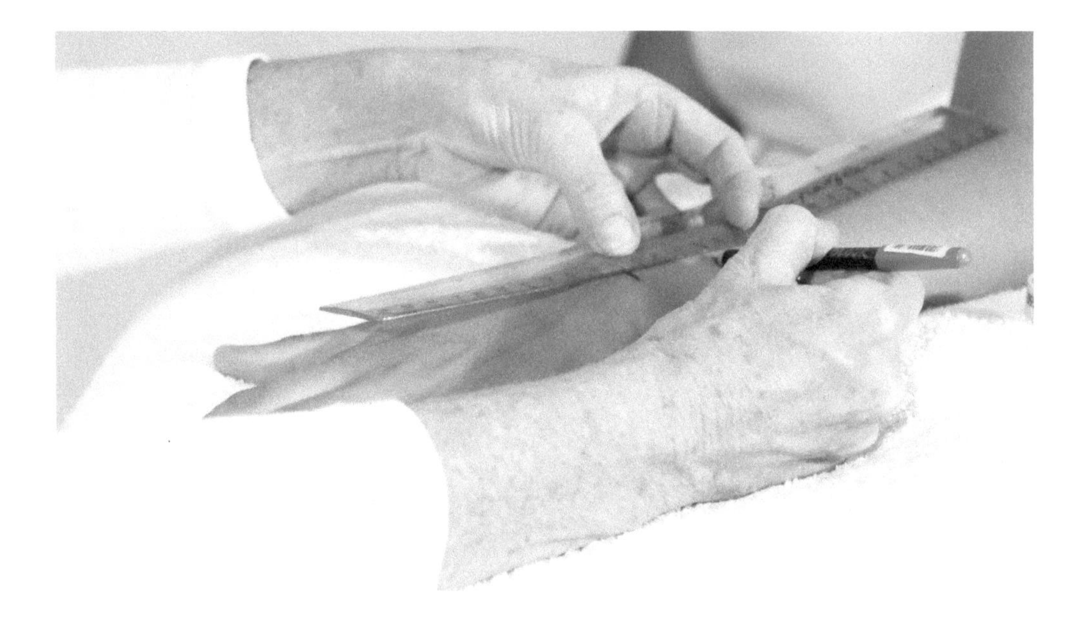

How to convert the circumference measurements into volume

The volume of each cylinder is worked out separately using a mathematical formula for a cylinder, 4cm in height and the measurement of the circumference.

Formula: Volume = Circumference^2 divided by pi (pi = 3.142)

$$V = \frac{Circumference^2}{\pi}$$

In simple terms if the circumference is, for example, 15.2cm the sum looks like this

15.2 x 15.2 = 231.04 / (divided by) π 3.142 = 73.54ml

Repeat this sum with the circumference for each 4cm section.

The volume of each cylinder is added together to calculate the cylindrical volume of the whole arm. Do this separately for both arms.

To calculate the amount of swelling, subtract the total sum of the non-swollen arm from the total sum of the swollen arm and the difference is the fluid volume of the lymphoedema.

Once you have the before and after volume figures for each arm, further calculations can be done to express the difference as a percentage in relation to the normal arm.

The mathematical formula for this is 100 divided by the volume of the normal arm multiplied by the difference.

Results are expressed as percentage excess volume of the swollen arm compared to the normal arm.

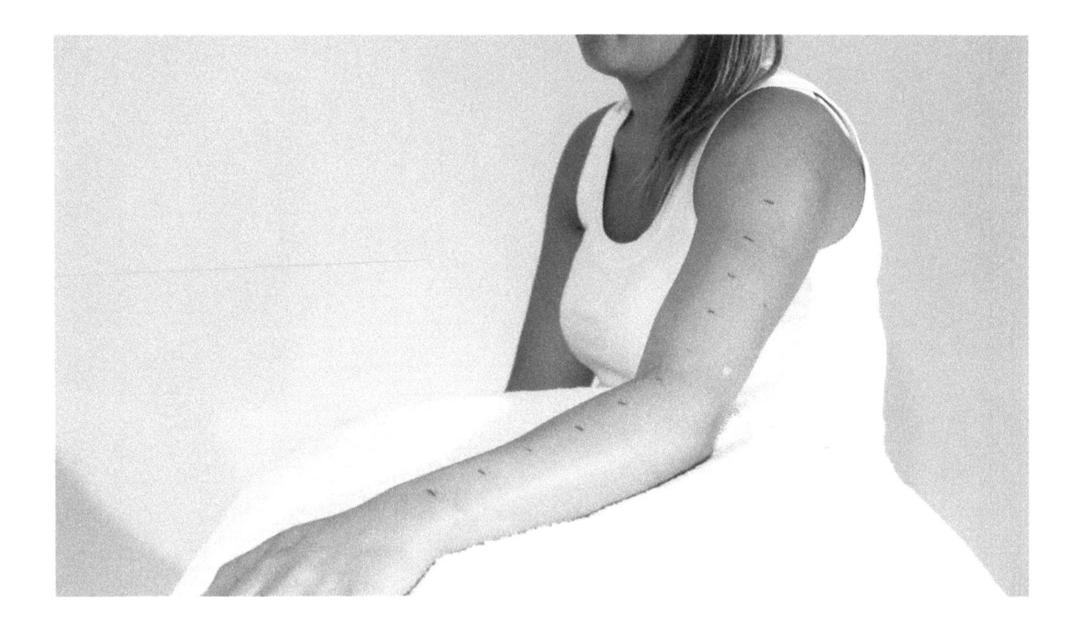

In the next chapter you will be able to take a closer look at the data sets for each of the cases that were first introduced in Chapter 2, Small Steps to Research.

Reflection

- The circumference of each 4cm cylinder of the arm is measured
- A simple mathematical formula is used to calculate the volume of each cylinder
- Be inspired by the results and rise up to the tape measure challenge! You can do this

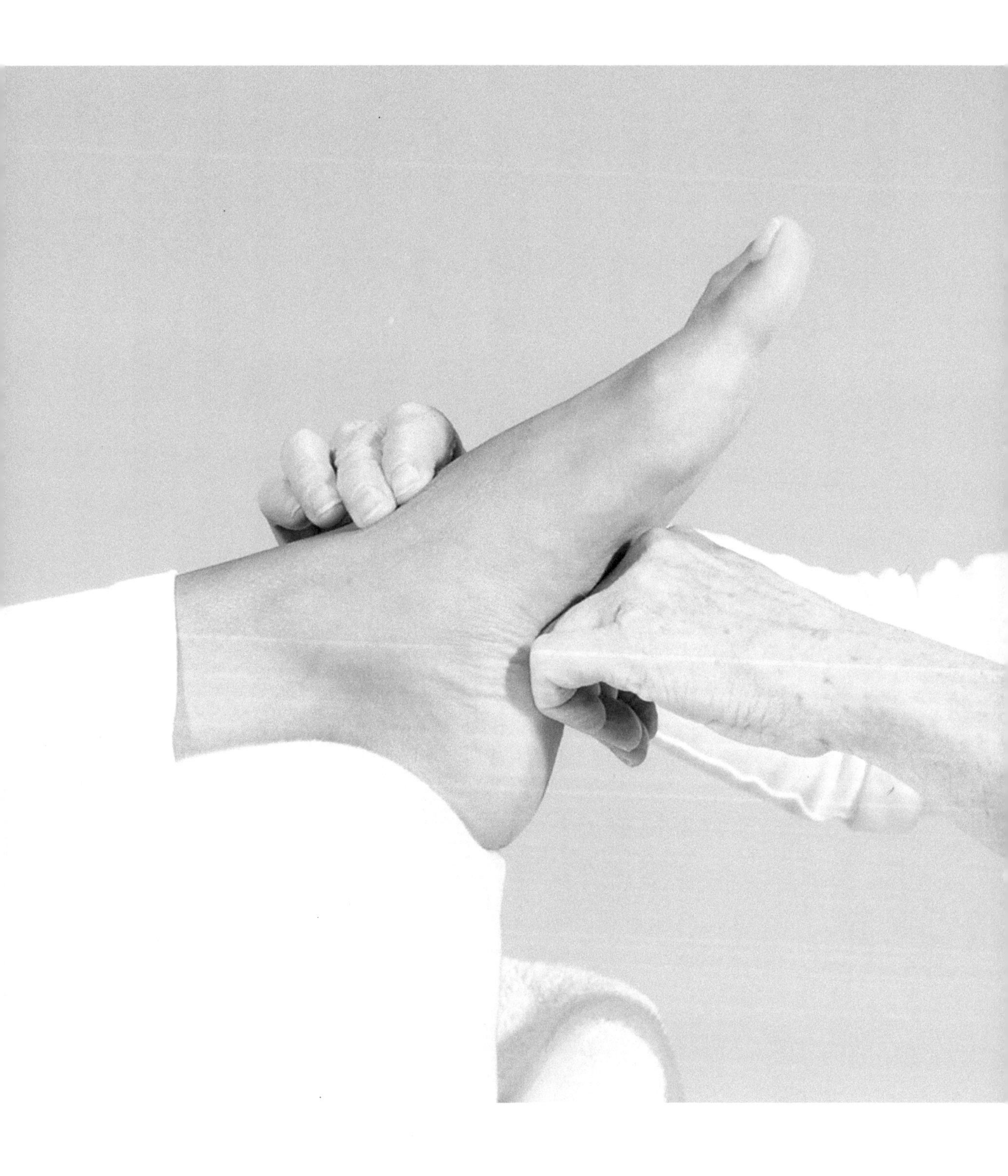

Chapter 9
Data and Research

Expectation

In this chapter discover how compelling the facts and figures are when they are organised into individual data sets, now that you know how to measure and what the calculations mean. You will be able to read a summary of the published RLD research studies and find out more about the formulaic way a research abstract is written. Ultimately the first small study is the foundation and subsequent research publications form the building blocks of an evidence base.

In the following research case studies, first introduced in Chapter 2, each case acts as its own control. The swollen arm is compared to the normal arm before and after RLD. Each case is similar and collectively they are a case series.

Together these six cases are the first small step, a building block in the foundation for the future of RLD research. The first abstract is about this study.

A research abstract is a concise summary of a study, written in a formulaic way. The title explains what the study is about. The background is a summary of the literature review and forms the hypothesis for the research. The method sums up how the study was done. The results and conclusion form the rationale for further research. The second and third abstracts are from subsequent published RLD research.

All measurements and calculations in the research were done using this method of LVCM, detailed in the previous chapter.

Participant 1

Jane is a 62-year-old who had lymphoedema for seven years in her right arm, her dominant side.

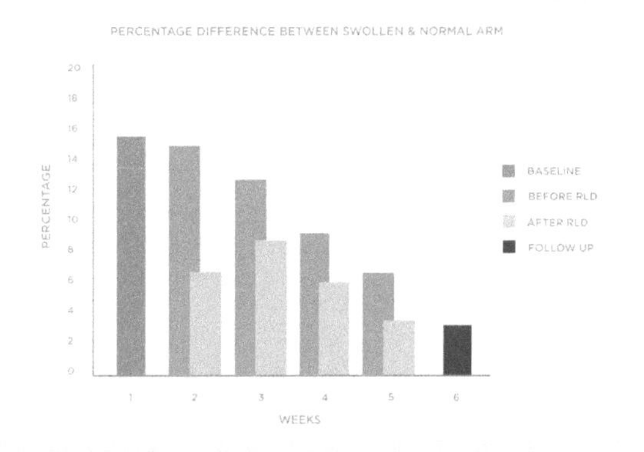

Chart 02: **Percentage difference between swollen & normal arm**

At baseline, the proximal section of the swollen arm was 16% bigger, and the distal 14.4% bigger. This meant the arm was 15.4% bigger than the unaffected left arm and it contained 358.96ml.

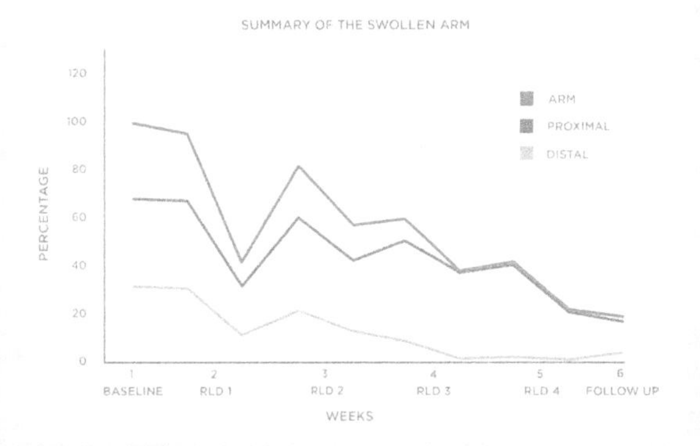

Chart 03: **Summary of the swollen arm**

From baseline week 1 to follow-up week 6, Jane lost 289.34ml from 358.96ml (100%), which is 80.6% of the swelling (See chart 3). Her right arm went from 15.4% bigger than the normal arm to only 3% (See Chart 02).

The ratio of volume change was greater in the distal section of the arm during RLD 1 & 2 and proximal during RLD 3 & 4. After RLD 3, the distal volume was reduced to normal and the remaining excess is proximal (See Chart 04).

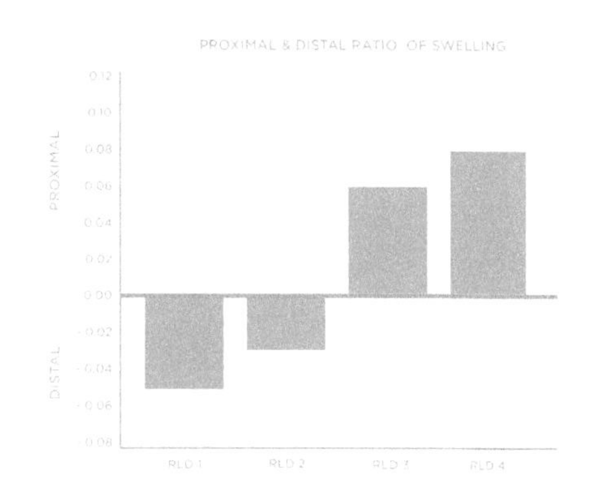

Chart 04: **Proximal & distal ratio of swelling**

MYCaW Concern 1, Swelling and 2, Aching. Baseline MYCaW scores indicate a negative trend, and at follow-up scores are positive. Results show a significant improvement for each concern (See Chart 05).

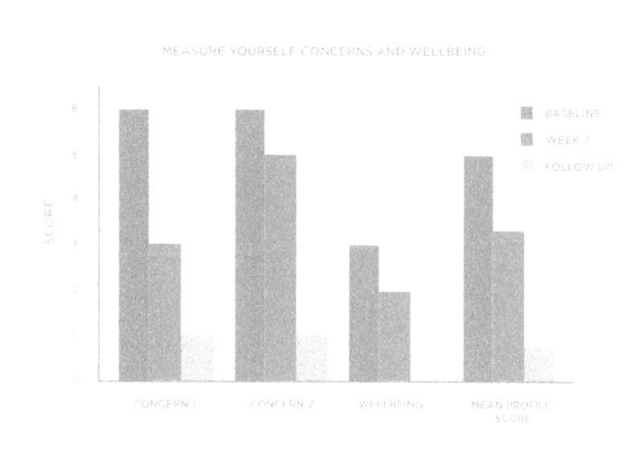

Chart 05: **MYCaW scores**

"My right arm is much lighter now. Prior to starting I had a lot of fluid at a pocket underarm and this too has lessened. Everything I struggled with, clothes, hobbies and driving are no longer a problem. Not embarrassed to take a long-sleeved cardigan off and wear short or sleeveless blouses, which has given me my confidence back." - Jane

Participant 2

Marie is a 53-year-old who had lymphoedema for three years in her dominant right arm, after a mastectomy and full axillary lymph node clearance.

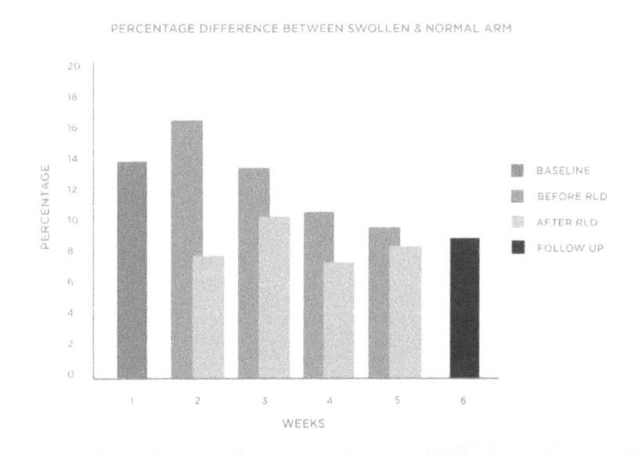

Chart 06: **Percentage difference between swollen & normal arm**

At baseline the proximal section of the swollen arm was 16.2% bigger and the distal 9.5% bigger. Overall the cylinder of her arm was 13.9% bigger than the normal arm and contained 366.78ml.

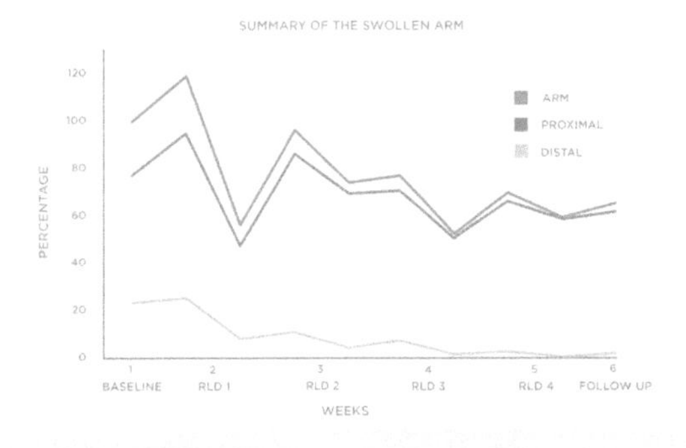

Chart 07: **Summary of the swollen arm**

From baseline week 1 to follow-up week 6, Marie lost a total of 132.06ml from 366.78ml (100%, 36% of the swelling) (See Chart 07). Her right arm went from 13.9% bigger than the normal arm to 8.9% (See Chart 06).

The ratio of volume change was greater in the proximal arm than distal during each RLD treatment and proximal excess greater than the distal. After the second RLD, the distal volume became normal, and the remaining excess is proximal (See Charts 07 & 08).

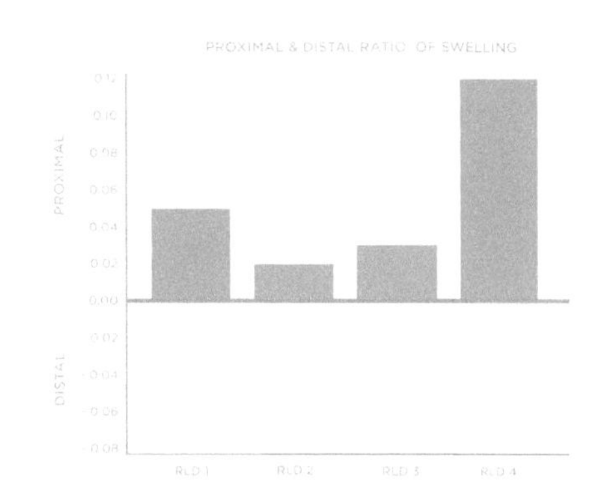

Chart 08: **Proximal & distal ratio of swelling**

MYCaW Concern 1, Swelling and 2, Aching. MYCaW Concern 1 score shows a negative trend. Week 3 and post-intervention are positive. The change in wellbeing is due to unrelated sad news. A reduction of 2 indicates a significant improvement. The greatest improvement was in Concern 1, "Swelling" (See Chart 09).

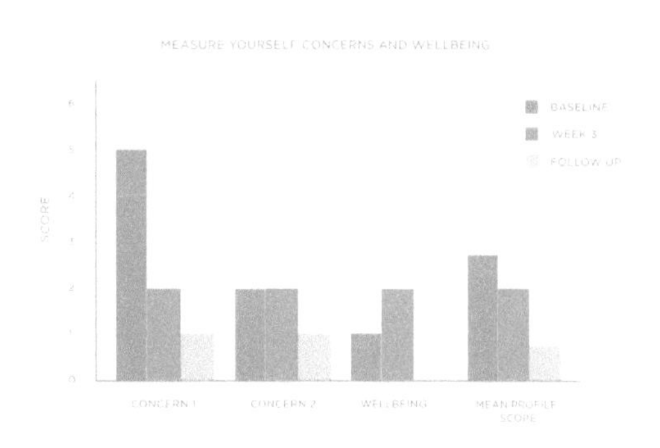

Chart 09: **MYCaW scores**

"It used to take me all day to do the ironing, I'd do a couple of things and stop because my arm was aching, now I've managed to get it all done without stopping." - Marie

Participant 3

Jean is a 38-year-old, who had lymphoedema in her dominant right arm for eight years, since a mastectomy, full axillary lymph node clearance and breast reconstruction surgery.

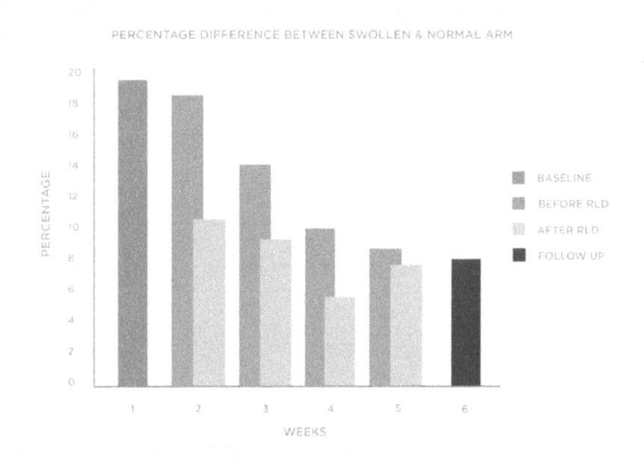

Chart 10: **Percentage difference between swollen & normal arm**

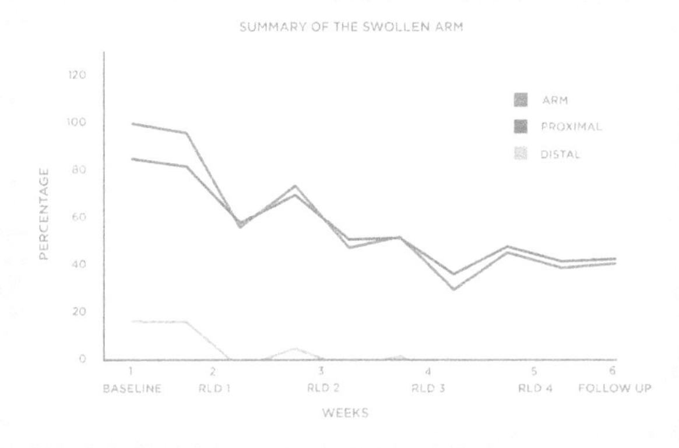

Chart 11: **Summary of swollen arm**

At baseline week 1, the proximal section of the swollen arm was 26.4% bigger, and distal was 8.1% bigger. Overall the cylinder of the arm was 19.5% bigger than the normal arm, with 456.97ml.

From baseline week 1 to follow-up week 6, Jean lost 270.25ml of 456.98ml (100%, 59.1%) (See Chart 11). Her right arm went from 19.5% to 7.9% bigger than the normal arm (See Chart 10).

The excess Jean had in the proximal section of the arm was greater than the distal section. After the first RLD treatment, distal volume reduced to normal, and the remaining excess was in the proximal arm (See Chart 12).

MYCaW Concern 1, Swelling and Concern 2, Aching.

MYCaW scores for Concern 1 Swelling, and 2, Aching, show a positive trend. The difference is greater than 2 which is a significant improvement. The wellbeing score was affected by news that Jean had to start another course of oral chemotherapy (See Chart 13).

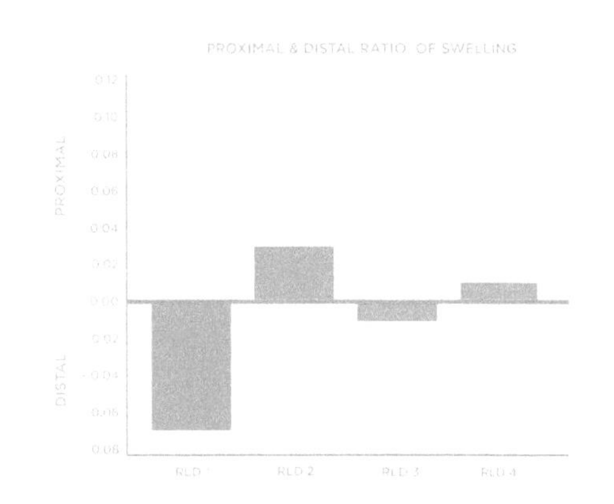

Chart 12: **Proximal & distal ratio of swelling**

After RLD 1 the swelling in her shoulder was much less, and Jean bought a new outfit, a size smaller! This area is above the measurable cylinder of the arm, and not included in the figures. She was so happy that she looked and felt radiant. A week later she joined a gym and started doing Zumba. Asked why she had not done this before, she replied, "I couldn't, because everyone would have been staring at my arm." A lovely example of reflexology, in this case RLD, helping to improve quality of life.

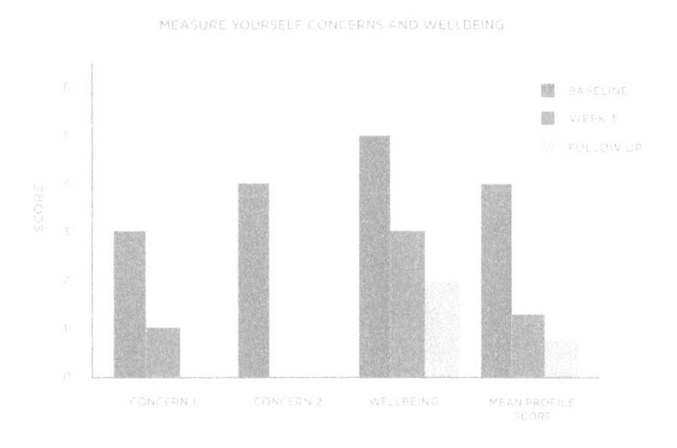

Chart 13: **MYCaW scores**

She sadly passed away peacefully at the end of 2015.

> *"Not having to go up an extra size is fab. Wearing tops that are not too tight on my one arm. I don't sit with my arm elevated so much anymore, which has been noticed by my family. I now go to Zumba classes and the gym. This has helped my confidence," said Jean.*

Participant 4

Carol is a 56-year-old who had lymphoedema for four years in her non-dominant left arm, since a mastectomy and full axillary lymph node clearance.

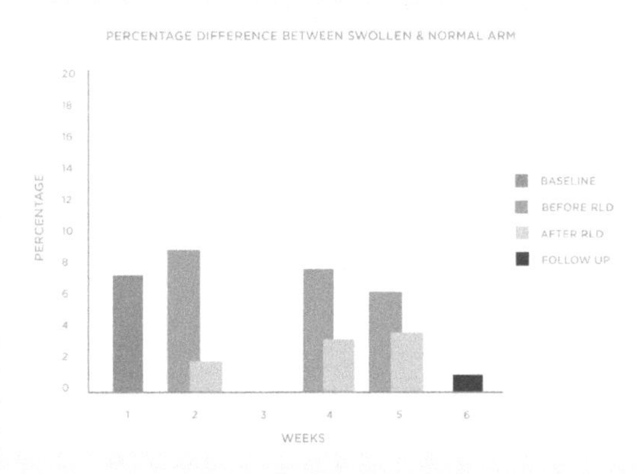

Chart 14: **Percentage difference between swollen & normal arm**

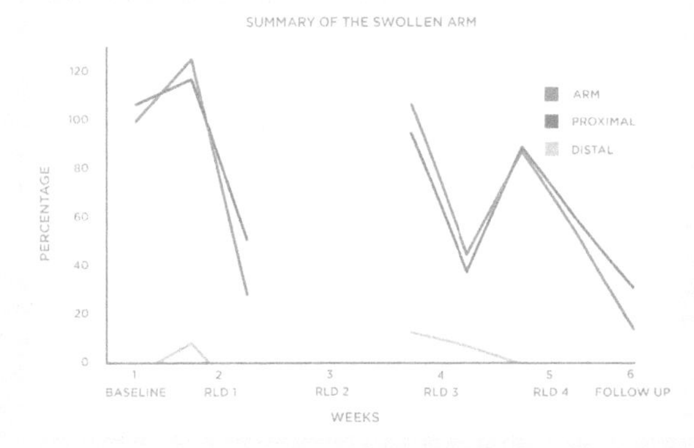

Chart 15: **Summary of the arm**

At baseline the proximal part of the swollen arm was 12.3% bigger and the distal -1.3% smaller. The arm was 7.1% bigger than the normal arm and contained 146.03ml.

Data for Carol is incomplete because she missed a week due to a last-minute holiday.

From baseline to follow-up Carol lost 126.53ml of 146.03ml, that is 86.6% of the excess (100%, 86.6%) (See Chart 15). Her left arm went from 7.1% bigger to only 0.9% (See Chart 14).

Carol had more proximal swelling than distal. At baseline all of the swelling was proximal. The distal section of the left arm was 1.3% smaller than the right dominant arm. There was a slight increase in swelling between baseline and RLD 1, and after this the distal volume reduced to normal (See Chart 16).

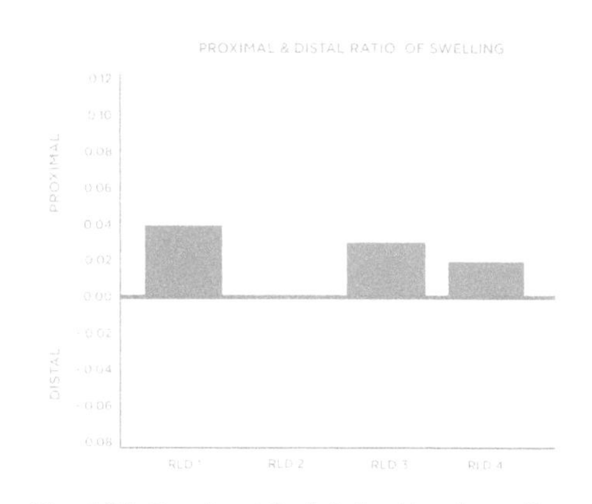

Chart 16: **Proximal & distal ratio of swelling**

The last-minute holiday involved a 5-hour flight each way. She felt so good after the first session and she did not wear compression on either flight. In spite of this the volume of swelling remained lower than at baseline, even after flying!

MYCaW Concern 1, Swelling and 2, Pain. Baseline MYCaW scores show a negative trend, and the post-intervention follow-up scores are positive (See Chart 17).

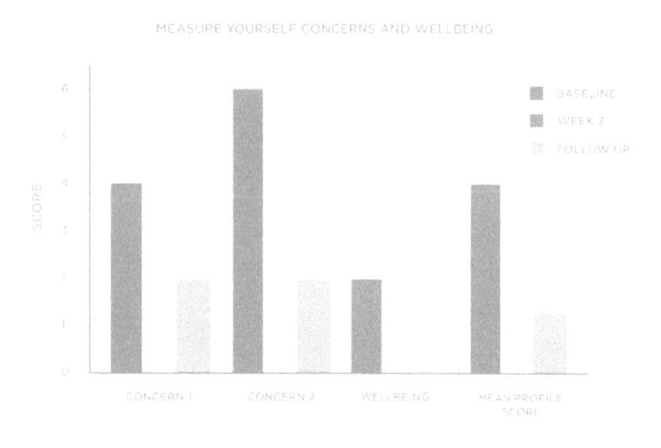

Chart 17: **MYCaW scores**

"Arm is a lot better. Lymph underarm felt like a tennis ball and I couldn't put my arm down comfortably, but this feels a lot better. My shoulder is much more mobile, a lot easier than it was, feels lighter, no bulges, feels normal." - Carol

Participant 5

Andrea is 48 years old and had lymphoedema for ten years in her left non-dominant arm since a lumpectomy and full axillary lymph node clearance.

At baseline week 1, the proximal section of the swollen arm was 13% bigger than the normal arm and the distal section, 31.1% bigger. Overall her left arm was 19.5% bigger and contained 456.98ml.

From baseline week 1, to follow-up week 6, Andrea lost 314.49ml of 456.98ml (100% - 74% of the excess) (See Chart 19). The difference between the arms went from 19.5% to only 5.1% (See Chart 18).

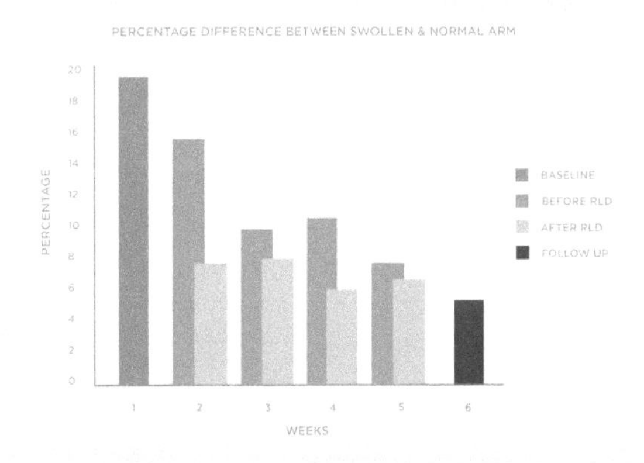

Chart 18: **Percentage difference between swollen & normal arm**

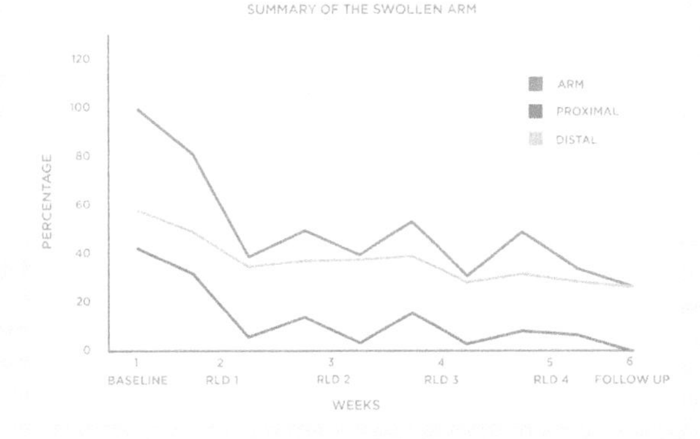

Chart 19: **Summary of swollen arm**

Distal swelling is greater than proximal throughout the study. At follow-up the proximal volume is normal, and the remaining excess swelling is in the distal section of the arm.

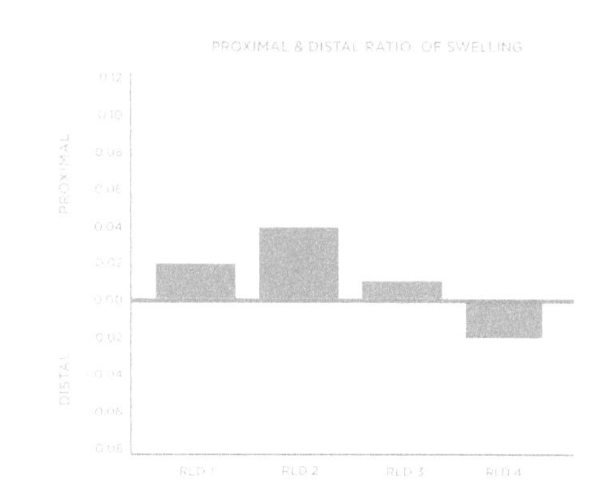

Chart 20: **Proximal & distal ratio of swelling**

The ratio of reduction in the arm volume was greater in the proximal part than the distal, during the first, second and third RLD treatment, and at the fourth treatment the ratio was greater in the distal section of the arm (See Chart 20).

MYCaW Concern 1, Cosmetic (she needed to wear a glove and half sleeve, compression garments which she hated the sight of), and 2, Aching.

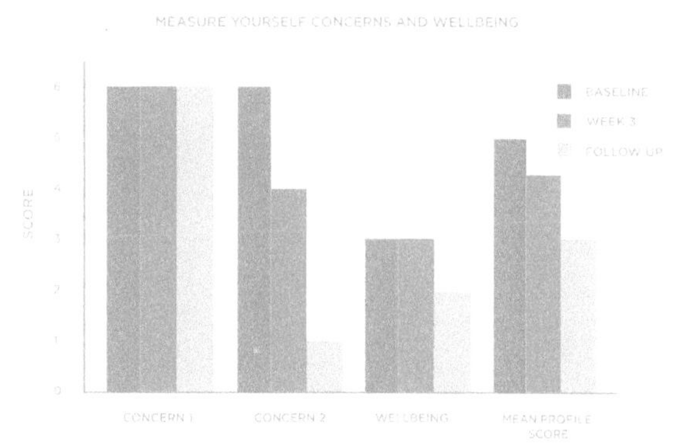

Chart 21: **MYCaW scores**

Baseline MYCaW scores show a negative trend. Concern 1 is unchanged, as Andrea still had to wear the sleeve and glove (See Chart 21).

"Having had my course of reflexology my left arm seems a lot lighter, also swelling seems to have reduced in size. Shoulder not aching, more flexible and moveable, swelling also reduced underarm. Fingers are more flexible, able now to grip objects and make a fist. I was unable to carry out these tasks before reflexology." - Andrea

Participant 6

Sian, 49 years old, had lymphoedema for five years in her right dominant arm since a lumpectomy and axillary lymph node clearance.

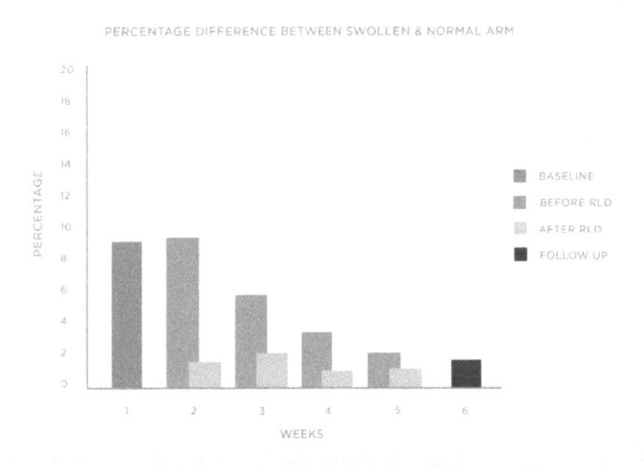

Chart 22: **Percentage difference between swollen & normal arm**

At baseline the proximal part of the swollen arm was 10.6% bigger than the other and the distal 5.9% bigger. The arm was 9.1% bigger and contained 322.09ml.

From baseline week 1, to follow-up week 6, Sian lost 270.67ml of 322.09ml (100%, 84%) (See Chart 23). The difference between arms went from 9.1% to only 1.5% (See Chart 22).

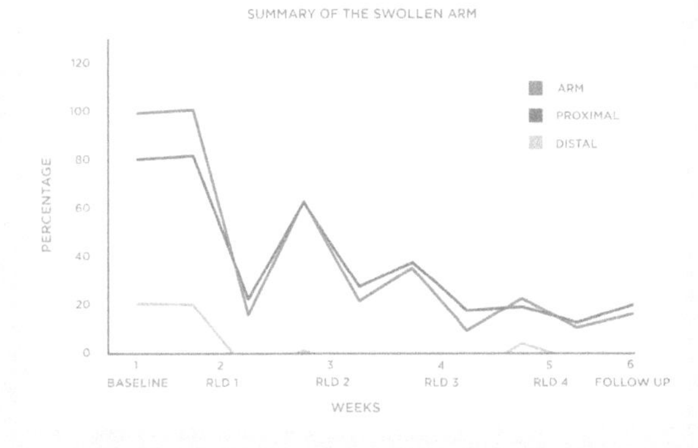

Chart 23: **Summary of swollen arm**

The proximal arm is holding most of the excess and after the first RLD treatment the volume of the distal section of the arm was the same size as the normal arm.

For Sian the ratio of reduction in arm volume was greater, distal during the first and fourth RLD and proximal during second and third treatment (See Chart 24).

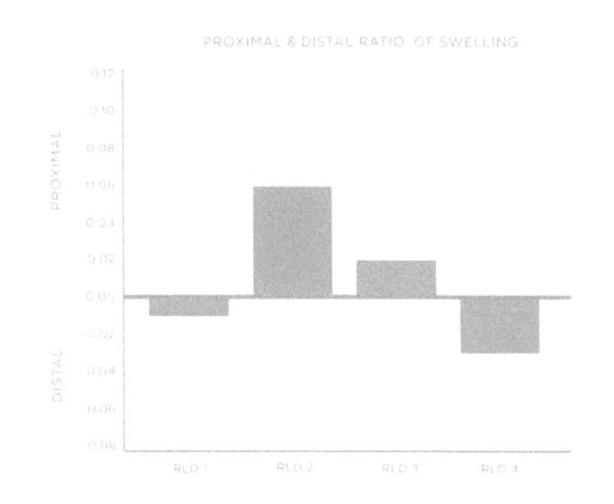

Chart 24: **Proximal & distal ratio of swelling**

MYCaW Concern 1, Swelling and Concern 2, Aching. Baseline MYCaW scores for Concern 1 & 2 show a negative trend and the wellbeing score is positive. The post-intervention follow-up scores are positive (See Chart 25). The reduction is greater than 2 for each profile, and this shows significant improvement.

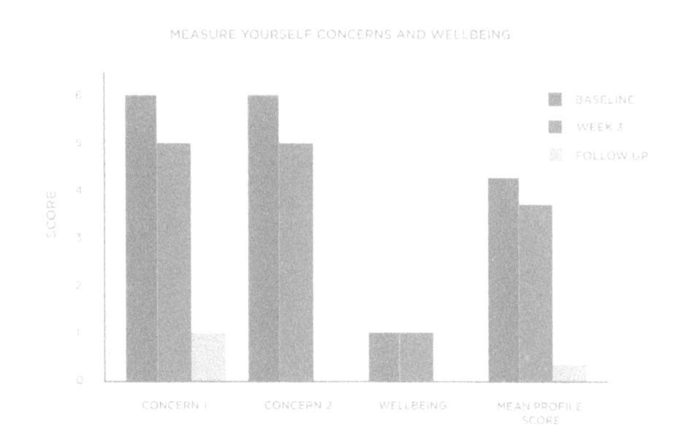

Chart 25: **MYCaW scores**

"I feel like I have my arm back, more able to do everyday tasks i.e. ironing. I feel good about myself and it has helped my confidence. The sleeves on my clothes feel looser. After this I don't want my arm to go back to how it was. I feel normal again. It has inspired me to do my exercises myself as I have got out of the habit. I had forgotten what it felt like to be normal again." - Sian

RLD research abstract 1

Reflexology for the management of secondary lymphoedema in patients affected by treatment for breast cancer: An exploratory study

Authors: Sally Kay, Judith Whatley, Philip Harris (*European Journal of Integrative Medicine* Volume 4, Issue 3, Pages e359–e360, Sept. 2012)

Background: Breast cancer is the most common cancer in the UK. Following medical intervention approximately 20% of breast cancer patients suffer lymphoedema. After breast cancer, a person may experience psychological or emotional difficulties due to altered body image, and a swollen limb can exacerbate this (Mackereth & Carter 2006). Research suggests that survivors with lymphoedema are more disabled, and they experience a poorer quality of life and more psychological distress than survivors without lymphoedema (Bernas et al. 2010, Pyszel et al. 2006, Ridner 2005). There is a need for more effective interventions and further research into a range of physical therapies for the management of lymphoedema. Reflexology is a physical therapy focusing on the feet. Practitioners use specific pressure with thumb, finger and hand techniques to stimulate these reflexes on the premise that this effects a physical change in the body. Anecdotally, cancer patients suffering from lymphoedema report positive effects on the swollen arm after reflexology treatment.

Aims and objectives: To explore the use of the RLD (Reflexology Lymph Drainage) technique as a precision treatment for the reduction of lymphoedema, swelling of the arm following treatment for breast cancer.

Method: As part of an undergraduate project, six participants with unilateral secondary lymphoedema were recruited from a South Wales cancer care organisation. The participants received four consecutive weekly Reflexology Lymph Drainage (RLD) treatments. Limb Volume Circumference Measurement (LVCM) was the primary outcome measure used. This method is widely used for calculating arm volume (NHS 2008). Measure Yourself Concerns and Wellbeing (MYCaW) was used to gather subjective data (Patterson et al. 2006). LVCM and MYCaW measures were taken at baseline, the intervention stage, and at follow-up (one week post-intervention).

Results: Positive trends were observed on both outcome measures for all six participants. As a group, the results indicated a statistically significant reduction in arm volume, from baseline to follow-up ($t=6.93$, $df=5$, $p=0.001$) on LVCM. MYCaW mean profile scores from baseline to follow-up also showed a significant improvement ($Z=-2.207$, $p=0.027$). The results were also supported by the qualitative data reported by participants.

Conclusion: Findings of this exploratory study suggest that RLD may be helpful in the management of secondary lymphoedema. A more robust research design is needed to test for a causal link between the application of reflexology and possible outcome benefits.

In 2013 on the strength of these initial findings, Welsh cancer charity Tenovus awarded funding of £12,263 for further RLD research, to be conducted in partnership with Cardiff Metropolitan University. The intervention phase was completed between January and June 2014.

From this study two research papers have been published. RLD abstract 2 is a quantitative paper and RLD abstract 3 is qualitative.

RLD research abstract 2

Use of reflexology in managing secondary lymphoedema for patients affected by treatments for breast cancer: a pilot study

Authors: Judith Whatley, Rachael Street, Sally Kay, Philip Harris (Published: *Complementary Therapies in Clinical Practice* Volume 23, May 2016, Pages 1–8)

Purpose: The aim of this feasibility study was to examine the use of Reflexology Lymph Drainage (RLD) in the treatment of breast cancer related lymphoedema (BCRL) with a view to further research.

Methods: An uncontrolled trial was conducted with 26 women who had developed lymphoedema in one arm following treatment for breast cancer. Changes in upper-limb volumes and in participant concerns and wellbeing were measured. Qualitative data were also collected.

Results: A significant reduction in the volume of the affected arm was identified at follow-up compared to baseline. This reduction in volume appeared to be maintained for more than six months. Participant concerns were significantly reduced and their wellbeing significantly increased. No serious adverse effects were reported.

Conclusions: RLD may be a useful intervention for BCRL although the results could not be attributed to the reflexology intervention because of research design limitations. The main conclusion was, however, that there was sufficient evidence for further research using a randomised controlled trial.

RLD research abstract 3

Experiences of breast cancer related lymphoedema and the use of reflexology for managing swelling: A qualitative study

Authors: Judith Whatley, Rachael Street, Sally Kay (Published: Complementary Therapies in Clinical Practice Volume 32, August 2018, Pages 123–129)

Background and purpose: An estimated 1 in 5 women surviving breast cancer will go on to develop breast cancer related lymphoedema (BCRL). There is a gap in the literature capturing experiences of people living with BCRL who use complementary therapies.

Materials and methods: Data were collected from 26 participants via a semi-structured interview. Questioning centred around their personal experiences of living with lymphoedema, and their use of Reflexology Lymph Drainage.

Results: Four main themes emerged which comprised physical and psychosocial impacts of lymphoedema, experiences of physical change, and the return of optimism. RLD treatment was considered pleasant and non-invasive, and the reduction in swelling helped with pain and mobility.

Conclusion: The main conclusion from this qualitative evaluation was that participants perceived benefit on physical and psychological levels. Participation in the study appeared to help re-engagement with normal life. Further research is needed to quantify the changes in these parameters.

The overall trend seen in these results shows similarities to those of the participants who took part in the first study.

Case studies and testimonials in the next chapter provide further anecdotal evidence about the infinite possibilities for RLD. The potential uses for this simple reflexology treatment are truly astonishing!

Reflection

- Presentation of organised data sets provides compelling evidence of the benefits of RLD that can be achieved
- A case series of six participants is the foundation for further RLD research
- A research abstract is a concise summary of a study

Section 5

THE RIPPLE EFFECT

Chapter 10
RLD Case Studies and Testimonials

Expectation

This chapter features a small sample of some of the many RLD case studies and the testimonials of others and illustrates the tangible benefits of RLD. Full permission has been given to publish the details providing a glimpse into the many therapeutic benefits and infinite possibilities of RLD as a non-invasive, pleasant and effective treatment.

As part of the RLD training, reflexologists are invited to submit a case study. On successful completion, the reflexologist's name and contact details are added to the Approved Therapists page on the RLD website, www.reflexologylymphdrainage.co.uk. Originally this was to help people with lymphoedema find an RLD trained reflexologist and to recognise and differentiate between RLD and a standard reflexology treatment, even though reflexology treatment has many benefits for patients affected by a cancer diagnosis.

Reflexology is becoming more accepted in hospice care, to help support patients who are affected by life limiting conditions, due to its well known benefits including relaxation. However, it is unlikely to focus on management of lymphoedema without specialist training in RLD.

The remarkable outcomes of RLD treatments have far exceeded the aim and all expectations in what started as an explorative treatment to help relieve some of the distressing side effects of lymphoedema. Instead it has organically evolved into something with the potential to change the perception of reflexology and make a positive difference to the lives of many people. The results of the published research are very promising, and will hopefully form the cornerstone of future studies, which will contribute to the understanding and integration of reflexology. This is supported by a growing database of case studies, which provide anecdotal evidence of some of these unexpected RLD results. This growing body of evidence has recurring themes to suggest that RLD has a positive effect on other non-cancer related auto-immune disorders and inflammatory conditions. The possibilities appear to be infinite!

A small sample of case studies along with a few extracts from others are featured in this chapter. Full permission has been given to publish the details. RLD case studies include a minimum of four treatments.

As far as I'm concerned, a good case study is an honest account of the end-to-end process. Very often it's the detail, the small things, that make all the difference to someone, and not necessarily one with a perfect set of results. One of my favourite recurring themes in many RLD case studies is the gift of **hope**. With no cure for lymphoedema, being diagnosed with it after breast cancer can be the final straw, and with no getting away from it, this can feel like a **hopeless** situation.

RLD is a pleasant and non-invasive treatment with the potential to make a positive difference and help to manage this debilitating condition. For the comfort of people who are self-conscious about body image after their surgery, there is no need to get undressed to receive RLD, only to remove shoes and socks. In turn all of this helps to improve self-confidence, quality of life and enable people to regain an element of control.

The hardest thing in this chapter is choosing from so many wonderful and varied examples. My grateful thanks go to everyone for sharing their RLD experiences.

In the first chapter of this book, I introduced Janet Le Sueur, MLD therapist, who I met at NACTHPC conference in 2012. Her words after hearing my presentation were, "...and now I want to learn reflexology so that I can access her course" (see page 38). Five years later Janet qualified as a reflexologist and attended RLD training in January 2017. Five years later this is her case study.

Case studies

Case study 1: Breast cancer related lymphoedema by Janet Le Sueur

Lisa is a 59-year-old female who is married, with two grown-up children and she supports her elderly frail parents. Lisa strives to be fit and healthy, and despite persistent pain and fatigue, she enjoys a weekly Pilates class and walks the dog every day. Lisa has a positive mental attitude towards lifestyle and wellbeing choices. She takes good care of herself and body image is important to her.

Medical history

In November 2003 Lisa had breast cancer surgery, a wide local excision & axillary node clearance and in February 2004 a skin sparing mastectomy with immediate reconstruction with latissimus dorsi flap and an implant. Eight years later the reconstruction was revised, the implant changed and scar tissue removed due to chronic pain. Lisa also suffers with fibromyalgia which causes aching muscles, brain fog, fatigue and poor sleep.

Lisa has previously had several intensive MLD therapy sessions with the local lymphoedema service and monthly follow-up appointments. She has tried Bowen therapy primarily to increase the range of movement, and found this helpful. She also has regular acupuncture to relieve her fibromyalgia symptoms.

Her presenting conditions are swelling of the left breast, trunk and around the elbow and upper arm. She has a persistent area of numbness and altered sensation under the left arm. Lisa suffers with varying degrees of chronic pain depending on her level of activity but does not like taking pain killers.

The aims and objectives for the treatment plan are to reduce swelling and pain with RLD by working three feet. Begin with the foot on the right unaffected side, then the left swollen side and repeat again on the right side. No adaptations to the protocol will be made.

Session 1. Lisa was intrigued by the underlying rationale and interested in the comparison with MLD. She has pain under the left axilla and in her elbow and the left arm feels weaker than the other side. Lisa had fallen and hurt her right hip and shoulder the previous week, she felt dreadful with the fibromyalgia pains, is tired all the time, suffering low mood and her sleep pattern is all over the place.

Lisa relaxed quickly only chatting to say how soothing she found it and how relaxed she felt. Immediate feedback was that both the pain and swelling were reduced and on standing she felt that the swelling under the axilla area was reduced and she felt "quite good". Also, her right hip was more flexible and looser with reduced pain.

The next day she reported she had an "odd feeling" in her left breast overnight and some tingling in the arm.

Janet: "If I had been doing MLD I would have been pleased with the outcome."

Session 2. Measurements were up slightly but not to pre-treatment level. We discussed how difficult it is to judge the swelling in the axilla & trunk area, and she realised she had been doing her bra up on a tighter hook! Lisa sent a text message the next day. Her armpit was "a bit sore" but not feeling full and her bra was on a tighter hook. She also had more energy.

Session 3. Lisa felt the pain had been better and more stable, but during the last few days had felt the breast & trunk pain again. However she had been wearing a memory foam bra and wondered if this was the cause. Measurements showed the volume loss had been maintained. Lisa sent a text message again the next day to say she had slept all night, which was almost unheard of for her, and felt much better!

Session 4. Lisa is pleased to say her bra remains on the smaller hook, the pain has been greatly reduced in the area under her arm. She also noticed a "fizzing" feeling, under the affected arm in the area of altered sensation post-operatively, but this settled. On the whole Lisa feels good, both pain and swelling is stable and reduced, generally she feels "quite well". Lisa feels there is an improvement and her arm is "good" and underarm only aches with certain movements.

Reflective practice

Self-evaluation: I have practised MLD for many years, which experience allows me to judge skin tension and tissue firmness and adjust the depth of movement and pressure to the individual. With RLD, working remotely, I do not have that feedback mechanism during the session. With MLD I can feel which pathways are draining better and adapt the treatment by repeating on an area, if required.

On a personal level, I like having a set sequence to follow, when learning something new. I learn best when what I am trying to achieve is presented clearly and with a scientific basis. I found it reassuring that Sally Kay's work did not conflict with MLD but gives an alternative way of expressing it. Due to my background, as a lymphoedema practitioner and MLD therapist, I found Sally's rationale fitted with my previous knowledge and experience.

What have I learnt? I had not expected such a rapid fluid loss, particularly from the breast & trunk areas. I was surprised that the loss was maintained over the week. I was delighted with the reduction of pain.

How does RLD differ from a more generic reflexology treatment? Firstly, the aims of the treatment are more specific. Prior to learning reflexology I had viewed it generally as merely "relaxing and balancing" but have grown to recognise that it can be so much more.

Potential uses for RLD

This case study has been insightful, it shows that even 14 years after breast cancer, it is still possible to effect a change. Compared with MLD, it is not intrusive to have a foot treatment, from a body image perspective. With conventional MLD, the massage is over the breast, chest and scar tissue, which some people might be reluctant to have, when a practitioner has to work in such intimate areas. With RLD I did not have to work directly over the wound area, which could be hypersensitive.

There can be a tendency to accept that the body might not fully restore after trauma surgery when a certain length of time has passed and this case study gives potential hope. I imagine I might use RLD as the core of the treatment and add further work to specific areas of concern. I am curious to know how this might work.

Conclusion

This case study involved a lady who has had longstanding BCRL and associated pain and swelling, particularly of the breast and axilla truncal area. It was challenging and intriguing. As "an expert patient", who has had many MLD sessions, I thought she would be able to make a good case study. As her oedema is longstanding and she has other health issues I was not sure if she would respond positively.

Overall the lymphoedema related pain and swelling were reduced. Unfortunately, due to her fibromyalgia there were other aches and pains, which she is aware fluctuate from day to day. Her sleep pattern has improved generally, with a whole night's sleep post treatment on one occasion. RLD was viewed as a preferred method due to the acceptable area of treatment and it being more relaxing and mainstream.

As a practitioner I was delighted with the outcomes in terms of volume difference. Whilst the limb related differential was small it was the truncal oedema that is so challenging to shift. The sequence is logical and easy to learn. I imagine in practice I could add this to a slightly longer sequence for this lady as well as working on areas for relaxation and other areas of pain.

I chose Janet's case study as she is an experienced MLD therapist, who trained in reflexology in order to learn RLD. This case is an existing client who has had MLD massage, and other complementary therapies, and her experience of these interventions provides an insight into the results of RLD. Best of all there is **hope** in this case study.

Case study 2: Palliative case study by Carol-Ann Barrett

When Sally requested case studies for inclusion in her book the hardest task was which to choose as now there are so many.

I first qualified as a lymphoedema therapist in 2001. However I am also a reflexologist and when I read an article on RLD I immediately contacted Sally. On our RLD training course one delegate had lymphoedema so was chosen as the model. This allowed for both immediate objective and subjective outcomes which were very positive. I immediately set about undertaking the case studies for the qualification. I also decided to conduct my own small clinical trial along the same protocol as Sally had done for the secondary arm lymphoedema, only I chose lower limb. Although small the results are also statistically significant.

A terminally ill patient with a gross secondary unilateral lymphoedema was referred to me for palliative MLD. This lady had been through a torrid time of allopathic treatment in the hope of some regression of the cancer. The treatments and lymph node resection that had resulted in the lymphoedema had sadly no impact on the cancer and the growths continued to ravage her body. When she came into clinic with her daughter the pain and discomfort was etched on her face. She was no longer able to wear shoes and her oedematous foot hung over a distorted slipper. She was groggy from pain relief and morphine.

I examined her leg and listened intently to her recounting the journey that had led her to my clinic. As she spoke her daughter wiped away a tear. She also looked exhausted and helpless, desperate for anything to relieve her mother's agony. Her limb was solid, a positive Stemmer's sign, and she was unable to flex her knee.

Once comfortable on the plinth I decided to do RLD. With the pressure of the lesions in the pelvis and groin and resection of the inguinal lymph nodes, I felt a contralateral drainage route for MLD would be compromised. I had hypothesised in my RLD treatments that whilst MLD exerted an epifascial push on the initial lymphatics and by inertia could activate deeper drainage pathways, I felt that RLD was having a deeper suctioning effect. During treatments patients would comment that they could feel the lymph draining from their limbs.

As I worked judiciously on this patient she started to drift in and out of a gentle slumber. I looked over to her daughter who smiled back with a look of amazement on her face as she saw the oedema in her mother's foot reducing before her eyes. At the end of the session her mother reported that she no longer felt pain in her pelvis. When she came to put her foot into the slipper she announced in excitement that her slipper was now too big for her foot. She looked younger in years with an incredulous smile on her face as if I had performed some sort of magic. It was magic and the capacity for the body to respond in such a powerful way to such gentle touch never ceases to amaze me!

As she had been my last patient that day I rang the daughter the next morning to enquire how the mother was. The daughter informed me that her mother had dozed in her chair most of the evening, had slept all through the night, something that she had not done for a while, and had not needed any pain relief or breakthrough pain medication. She had just woken, was smiling and asking when her next session was.

I had the privilege of treating this lady on two further occasions before she passed away. Her daughter was grateful that her mother had been helped in such a positive way.

The positive ripple effect of RLD stands out in this case study. Carol-Ann used RLD to help the patient who was suffering greatly. This was distressing for her daughter who looked exhausted and helpless, and was desperate for anything to relieve her mother's agony. She was able to see the relief her mum experienced receiving RLD from Carol-Ann.

Case study 3: Secondary lymphoedema, post-operative inflammation and pain case study by Carol-Ann Barrett

Another case that springs to mind was a lady with secondary arm lymphoedema on a maintenance programme of MLD, who required surgery on her lumbar spine. Following the decompression surgery she developed complications resulting in a drop foot which prevented her from walking properly. She also reported a complete loss of sensation in her left foot and severe neurological pain in her leg and groin. She was also unable to rise onto tiptoes or splay her toes. She was weary of being in pain and having been back and forth to the GP, hospital and specialist with no one offering her any solutions other than increasing her pain medication and re-scanning.

When she came to see me there was no oedema to the leg or foot. However in formulating a treatment plan I decided to try RLD on the basis that I would be able to reduce the lymphoedema in the arm whilst at the same time feeling confident that the Reflexology Lymph Drainage would be helpful with the post-operative inflammation. I was intrigued to see if this powerful intervention would ameliorate some of her iatrogenic neurological symptoms.

She agreed to weekly sessions and even after the first session she reported subjective positive outcome measures in reduced pain. As the treatments continued she was able to stand on tiptoes and splay her toes. She also reported a reduced burning sensation that had been so debilitating and had prevented her from sleeping at night, for which she had been prescribed amitriptyline.

The pain lessened to the extent that she was able to reduce her pain medication. After eight sessions of RLD she returned to the specialist. I was copied in to the letter from her specialist to her GP, and the final paragraph read: *"I am delighted that she feels that the operation has been beneficial now but I suspect this is due to a lot of hard work on the behalf of Carol-Ann Barrett as well."*

Recognition in writing from the medical profession that a complementary therapy has been effective is a rather rare occurrence and testament to the efficacy of RLD, not only in cases of lymphoedema but, as trained RLD therapists are finding and reporting, the applications of this therapy goes much further in alleviating many symptoms in a variety of other conditions.

Carol-Ann and Janet are both MLD therapists as well as reflexologists, and with their professional expertise and in-depth knowledge of working with the lymphatic system they had a choice of therapeutic approach to best suit the individual. Wonderful results for RLD!

Case study 4: Bartholin's cyst case study by Karen Kearney

Sarah is a 28-year-old who is generally fit and healthy. She was diagnosed with a Bartholin's cyst, which she described as "quite big and solid. It makes walking uncomfortable and intercourse impossible!" Her GP prescribed three courses of antibiotics, with little or no improvement. The GP said nothing else could be done until it got bad enough to need surgery.

It was following this that she started to see me for regular reflexology and the bonus was that I had just completed the RLD course.

Aims and objectives: To alleviate some of the discomfort by possibly reducing the size of the cyst. Use the RLD protocol for lower limb and with specific attention to the lower lymphatic reflexes.

Treatment plan: A course of four treatments, but for my own curiosity I did five, as she felt most of the positive results happened after the third treatment.

Treatment outcome: Amazing results! The cyst went from a "solid golf ball" to a "squidgy soft lump". The pain went completely and she was able to do normal everyday things without discomfort, including painless intercourse.

> *Client feedback: "I want to begin by just saying – oh my goodness, I just can't believe it! After being poked and prodded and having had test after test and then being told by my consultant there was nothing that could be done about my Bartholin's cyst (unless I basically became unable to walk!) I was really at my wits' end. Not only was I in pain most of the time, with very painful periods too, I was beginning to feel very depressed and low about the whole thing – then I was introduced to Karen who said she'd just done some training and perhaps it might help to have some Reflexology Lymph Drainage. I was a little sceptical, although I am a fan of complementary therapies, but had nothing to lose, so we went ahead and had five sessions from Karen. The first couple of sessions were very relaxing and I felt a little tingling in the area during*

treatment, but it was the third session that really made a difference and each session following that I not only began to see and feel the difference in the cyst, I was also feeling so much better mentally! Thanks to this treatment I am now pain free, and the cyst is tiny and soft. My periods are less painful, and my mood swings pre-menstrual are just a memory! I will definitely continue to see Karen on a regular basis - I now call her 'The Lady with the Healing Hands!' - Although she has clearly explained the healing comes from me, she just encourages the body to balance itself."

Case study 5: Breast cancer related lymphoedema of the arm case study by J. Williams

Jane is 56 years old, and six years ago she was diagnosed with a fast growing aggressive tumour in her left breast. She had 12 doses of chemotherapy to shrink the tumour before full mastectomy surgery. Post surgery, Jane was given six doses of radiotherapy and a year's treatment of Herceptin at the local oncology unit.

Jane's main problems were chronic fatigue and a hard sac of fluid the size of a golf ball under her left arm making her feel unbalanced, uncomfortable and self-conscious. Jane also reported a fluid-filled scar line. She described her overwhelming emotion as one of sadness that this was the result of surgery.

After four RLD sessions this is her feedback:

> *"Following surgery for breast cancer in 2010, I developed side effects which included swelling to my left upper arm and to the left side of my body. I was very conscious of this and it made my whole body feel unbalanced. I also had poor lymphatic drainage in the left underarm area which resulted in a hard lump the size of a golf ball in my left armpit which I would have to manually massage to assist drainage. Since undertaking the course of Reflexology Lymph Drainage treatments the swelling on my left side has gone and my body now feels in balance. The lump in my left armpit has not returned. The treatment has made a huge difference to my self-esteem as I feel more positive about my body."*

Conclusion: Overall this has been a very successful series of treatments and the client is completely satisfied with no recurrence of lymphoedema under her arm and marked improvement over the operation site.

Case study 6: Psoriatic arthritis case study by D. Stone

Dawn is 44 years old, and currently unable to work due to ill health. She was diagnosed with psoriatic arthritis many years ago and suffers greatly with very painful joints, psoriasis patches on her body, and both her legs are very swollen, in the knees and ankles. She also suffers with insomnia. Dawn had not tried reflexology before and was sceptical. After the first session, we were both amazed at the difference in her leg measurements. You could actually see the difference in her knees!

After the first session Dawn slept for 20 hours, the most sleep she had in years. She felt energised and did some chores she had not had the energy to do previously. By the end of the course of four treatments she was amazed by how quickly she felt relaxed and how much she slept after a treatment. She enjoyed her new energy levels and the fact that she had kneecaps again. She claims the weight loss was connected to the RLD as she did not change anything else in her lifestyle. She is no longer a reflexology sceptic!

Conclusion: I was amazed at the actual results of the RLD, such a visible difference in the size of her legs, from the first treatment to the last treatment. With the reduction in swelling, pain was not as bad nor was she as stressed. Her sleeping patterns and energy levels improved greatly and her general wellbeing was much better.

Many RLD case studies and clients often refer to weight loss as a treatment outcome. There is a case to be answered here, if RLD stimulates lymphatic drainage and the evidence points to this, maybe it is causing an effect on the lymphatic function in relation to the digestion and elimination of fats. It is also likely that as people begin to feel better physically and in themselves, they are more active and less inclined to comfort eat. Who knows? Either way, it's all good!

In the client feedback in case studies 4, 5 & 6 all confess to being sceptical before RLD. This reminds me how much I love to work with a sceptic. There is absolutely nothing to lose and everything to gain. It's a win-win!

The next case study is from another reflexologist who is also a lymphoedema therapist.

Case study 7: Lower limb swelling case study by Melanie Jeeves

Sue is a 57-year-old teacher who contacted me for reflexology. I saw her last year when she had Manual Lymphatic Drainage for bilateral lower limb swelling. At the time she was experiencing some difficulty in breathing and thought she had a chest infection. This was subsequently diagnosed as a collapsed lung and further investigations identified fluid on her lung and a benign tumour.

I was not prepared to proceed with MLD at the time because of her compromised breathing. However, as she was in some discomfort I offered her some light touch reflexology to see if it eased the symptoms and was advised that it did. She contacted me again this year following a road traffic accident, a head-on collision that had caused a fractured pelvis. During hospitalisation she had been provided with below knee DVT stockings and her legs had become swollen. She was finding it very difficult to flex her ankles and to bend her knee and was very upset by their appearance.

Sue is exceptionally thin and her GP had always thought her borderline anorexic and suggested that her low weight may have contributed to her swollen legs due to protein deficiency. Later last year this developed to the extent that she developed what sounds from her description to be lymphorrhoea, where the fluid oozes through the pores so much that when out, her shoes had filled up, which was clearly very distressing and frightening. This had not been investigated further and she had not been referred to the specialist lymphoedema clinic.

On this visit she was very low in mood and felt the accident had exacerbated her lower limb swelling. On examination oedema was palpable to the dorsum of both feet and present around the ankle and knee joints. Her limbs feel "fluidy" but she is very thin so the lymphoedema is more obvious. I explained the treatment and advised her that I will be taking measurements pre and post treatment to observe changes and monitor the effect of the treatment. Sue is having difficulty donning her tights, and compression garments would not be appropriate and may have a negative psychosocial impact in terms of body image.

The aim is to provide four sessions initially. The objective is to reduce overall limb swelling bilaterally and increase range of movement and mobility. It is hoped that the client will also begin to feel more positive and will be able to discuss any concerns should they arise on a weekly basis. Progress will be monitored and if there is no improvement alternative treatment options would be considered, such as referral to the Lymphoedema Clinic, hosiery and Simple Lymphatic Drainage.

Assessment and observations: There was no evidence of Stemmer's sign to toes. Pitting oedema to left and right dorsum of foot. Both calves felt "fluidy" and there was swelling on both knees and behind the knee at the popliteal lymph nodes. Thighs feel "fluidy", but there is no evidence of fibrosis. Limbs are warm to touch, no discolouration, skin changes or lymphorrhoea. The tissue does not feel taut although I am advised that when she was in hospital the tissue in her legs did become taut and she felt it was starting to happen again, which is why she contacted me.

Outcome measure: Measure Your Self Concerns and Wellbeing (MYCaW)
Concern 1 – discomfort
Concern 2 – appearance
Both rated at a 6 – "bothers me greatly"
Wellbeing – feeling very low, fearful that her legs will swell further, low body image

Post treatment there is immediate evidence of a reduction in swelling to the dorsum of both feet. The swelling has also reduced around the ankles and when she stood up she was able to flex her foot which was difficult prior to treatment. Sue seemed very positive and is delighted with the effects already.

Following last week's treatment during the evening the client had some discomfort in her right groin which eased overnight and disappeared by the following day. The oedema to the dorsum of both feet and around the ankles has reduced. Measurements indicate that the drainage is occurring primarily from the distal regions as the fluid is drained from these to the proximal region as would occur during Manual Lymphatic Drainage. The right leg, which had been uncomfortable at the inguinal area for the first night post treatment, has seen the greatest loss at 206.93ml. The left leg saw a slight gain of 23.25ml. The accumulative volume loss bilaterally now exceeds two litres after the third treatment. Sue is very pleased with the results as her mobility has improved, and she is less reliant on her crutches.

Both left ankle and both knees are now clearly defined with only slight palpable swelling to dorsum of right foot. Bilaterally at the knee there has been a reduction of 4cm (r leg) and 3cm (l leg). There have been no further episodes of groin pain. Over the course of the week both legs have reduced bilaterally, combined total more than 600mls, suggesting RLD is proving valuable both during and post treatment. The accumulative volume loss for the right leg now stands at 1708.09ml. and the left leg at 1322.86ml. A combined loss of more than three litres!

The client is understandably thrilled with the results! "I have knees" was the comment that greeted me today, as both are now clearly defined. Sue is finding that her mobility is improving all the time, and she has greater flexibility in her ankle and knee joints, which were so swollen and tight when we started. Sue is more positive in her outlook because she can see and feel the difference.

The final volume loss from the first treatment was as follows:
Right leg on first measurement, 6039.99ml, post sixth treatment 4002.86ml (total loss 2037.13ml)
Left leg on first measurement, 5877.49ml, post sixth treatment 4149.06ml (total loss 1728.43ml)
Combined volume loss bilaterally 3765.56ml

In conclusion: A wonderful outcome for Sue, who is a very slight build. Even small quantities of excess fluid on someone who has a slight frame feel exceptionally unpleasant. The aims and outcome have been achieved and psychologically Sue is a changed person, excited by the good results, and "happy to have her legs back". She is no longer using her crutches. MYCaW score is now 1.

Client feedback

> *"I had been suffering with uncomfortably swollen legs and ankles for two years. The doctors just put it down to the heat or having been standing for too long. However, my legs were swollen as much in the morning as at night, summer and winter. It got so bad I couldn't wear some of my slim fit legged trousers or get my feet into my shoes. It was seriously hindering my walking and movement and causing me a great deal of discomfort and distress. Luckily I was put in touch with Melanie and six treatments later I have my feet, ankles and knees back and she has drained over three litres of fluid. I am so grateful and cannot recommend the lymphatic reflexology highly enough." – Sue*

Reflective practice: I have been a lymphoedema practitioner since 2009 and a reflexologist since 2007. Unlike standard reflexology, RLD only targets the reflexes that are specific to the lymphatic system and thus it is possible to relate the outcome to the treatment. What I like about this therapy compared with MLD is the way it works with the body's lymphatic system and not trying to physically push the fluid to the lymph nodes. It is done at the body's own pace. I feel something deeper is occurring, and more natural healing process from within. MLD appears to have a positive effect initially, but then requires bandaging or a compression garment to hold the effect. For this lady there has been no bandaging and no garments to sustain the impressive results.

As a treatment, because of the gentle way RLD works, I feel it may be a safer gentler option. It can be beneficial for those who are palliative, helping without putting too much pressure on the body's systems. I have used this with good effect on a number of palliative patients and it has alleviated distress without overloading their already weakened systems.

I think that the potential for RLD as a treatment is endless. I am now trialling this with a lady who has lipoedema. Her alternative option is liposuction which is invasive. This has already seen a reduction in two weeks of treatments!

Case study 8: Breast cancer related lymphoedema case study by Cécile Rainsford

This case study was written as a blog for the Brave Ladies website, which specialises in post mastectomy swimwear, when one of the brave ladies found the confidence to model swimwear after a course of RLD. Here is her story.

In 1988, I was diagnosed with breast cancer and had surgery, chemotherapy and radiotherapy. This was successful but I was left with secondary lymphoedema swelling in my left arm, following breast cancer treatments.

Over the years, I have received various maintenance treatments and participated in a number of trials all aimed at curing and relieving the swelling. Nothing has worked, leaving me with excessive aches and pain in my neck and shoulder, a swollen heavy arm which I was unable to lift too high, the daily use of a support sleeve helping my arm not to swell too much, and the daily intake of antibiotics preventing me getting infections and an attack of cellulitis. Any slight injury to my skin can cause a serious infection which can take hold very quickly.

After almost 30 years of suffering with my arm, by chance I was invited to be part of a case study with Cécile Rainsford, a local trained reflexologist at Ped à Terre Reflexology who was taught by Sally Kay, the founder and researcher of Reflexology Lymph Drainage (RLD).

I received four RLD treatments with Cécile who measured my arm volume before and after each treatment which revealed a reduction of lymph fluid in my left arm. My left arm was initially 32% bigger than my non-swollen arm. Amazingly my arm has retained its reduced size after each treatment, and is now 20% bigger than my non-swollen arm. My arm can never be normal size again due to the removal of the lymph nodes but to regain a respectable shape and reduced size is astonishing and life changing.

I have continued to have reflexology sessions with my fantastic reflexologist, Cécile, as I find them so beneficial. Not only am I benefiting from relief in my arm but the reflexology is making a massive difference to my wellbeing and my immune system. The aches and pains in my neck and shoulder related to the treatment I had all those years ago have gone; my blood pressure has improved; the backache I suffer with has rescinded; my legs do not ache as much as they used to when I have been on my feet a lot due to my work; I can now lift my arm above my head; I am more relaxed and at ease with life in general.

The RLD treatment leaves you feeling totally relaxed and completely chilled out. The professionalism of Cécile, the ambience of the treatment room is perfect, and the ability to just totally relax during the treatment is wonderful. When the treatment is over, there is a feeling of being unable to move and 100% relaxed mood. My arm feels much lighter too.

I am so thankful to Cécile for making this possible and hope that the RLD research can continue for others suffering similarly, and to be a recognised treatment within the NHS and that the positive results can influence any medical specialists who deal with patients like me on a daily basis.

Thank you again to the wonderful work of Sally Kay and for Cécile Rainsford who has shown great passion in practising RLD.

Case study 9: Breast cancer related lymphoedema case study by Sally Kay

This case study began four years ago when Gail, a well-dressed, petite and attractive woman came to see me for RLD, after ten years of living with lymphoedema swelling. Despite being compliant with exercise, skin care and compression, her affected arm was 29.9% bigger than the unaffected side (see Fig. 39: Lymphoedema measurement sheet on page 208) - distal 47.3% bigger and proximal 18.1%, overall 29.9%, held 561.68ml). There were signs of fibrosis in the distal region, she had referred pain in the neck and shoulder, and swelling in the adjoining area of the trunk and in her hand.

Gail has the original RLD protocol and is measured each time she comes. At first the result pattern was consistent with the research case series (see Chart 01: Percentage of excess swelling between the swollen arm & the normal arm on page 53) but after six weeks the reduction slowed down. There is always a measurable loss and fluctuation between appointments, due to some of the usual suspects, hot weather, an episode of cellulitis, too much gardening! But the swelling quickly goes away again.

In this time she has blossomed and by her own admission, feels more like her old self.

RLD is the gift of **hope** in a previously hopeless situation. Gail has regained control of her life, lost weight, joined a gym and is able to wear her favourite clothes again.

> Some treatments for breast cancer can cause weight gain and in the complex minefield of emotional turmoil, the inevitable physical and psychological changes that go with the diagnosis and treatment, it can be notoriously difficult to lose afterwards.

At a recent appointment we compared the figures that day against her first visit, and reflected on the remarkable results and transformation. Her arm is only 4.2% bigger compared to 29.9%. The lymphoedema measurement sheet has all the details.

LYMPHOEDEMA MEASUREMENT SHEET No. Participant ID

Positioning for Measurement:

DATE		16th December 2014		25th October 2018			
		Right	Left	Right	Left	Right	Left
Circumference of hand							
DISTAL	1	18.3	16.3	16.7	16.1		
No. of cm from nailbed of middle finger / little finger (delete as appropriate) to head of ulna + 2cm = Then every 4 cm	2	21.9	19.3	19.3	18.7		
	3	27.3	22.5	21.9	21.4		
	4	30.7	24.3	25.2	24.1		
	5	31.9	25.6	26.5	25.9		
	6						
	7						
	8						
	9						
Distal segment vol.	10						
Difference R + L	ml	1120.42	760.85	785.68	738.00		
	ml/%	359.57	47.3%	47.68	6.5%		%
PROXIMAL							
	1	31.6	26.5	25.4	25.4		
	2	31.5	29.3	26.2	26.3		
	3	32.3	30.6	26.7	26.6		
	4	33.4	31.9	26.8	26.8		
	5						
	6						
	7						
	8						
Proximal segment vol.	9						
Difference R + L	10						
	ml	1320.88	1118.77	899.78	879.38		
	ml/%	202.11	18.1%	20.40	2.3%		%
Total limb volume	ml	2441.29	1879.62	1685.45	1617.37		
Difference R + L	ml/%	561.68	29.9%	68.08	4.2%		%
Shape segment ratio P:D							
Difference in P:D ratio							
+/- since last volume							
+/- since start of treatment							
%change in vol. since referral							

www.reflexologylymphdrainage.co.uk Sally Kay 2010

Fig. 39: Lymphoedema measurement sheet

Testimonials from reflexologists and clients

1. Gail Davies

The first testimonial is from the last case study, Gail

> *I was diagnosed with breast cancer in May 2003. This was followed by major surgery, removal of the lymph nodes, followed by 18 weeks of chemotherapy. Ten months later my arm started to swell and one morning I noticed my hand and fingers had swollen too.*
>
> *I contacted the hospital to explain what had happened and they informed me I had developed a condition known as lymphoedema. This condition was totally new to me and I didn't know what to expect or how it would affect my arm. I was referred to the lymphoedema service and began treatment with them. The lymphoedema nurses were very supportive and empathetic of the condition. Initially the appointments involved treatments such as massaging the arm, information and guidance on caring for the skin on your affected limb, and organising future appointments for check-ups.*
>
> *Over time my arm became very swollen, and I underwent the "48 hour bandaging treatment" which entailed layers of bandage and strapping being wrapped around your arm from fingertips to shoulder. This was very restrictive and by the end of the 48 hours was painful. Initially I experienced a reduction in the fluid but this would quickly revert back to its original shape after a few days. I was measured for a support garment. This consists of a long bandage in the guise of a very long glove which extends from the fingers to the shoulder. This is worn every day and removed at night.*

Over the years this support garment and treatment administered by the lymphoedema nursing staff helped however I was still unable to wear jackets, or garments which had narrow sleeves. I found this distressing and uncomfortable. I had to re-think the type of clothing I could wear on a daily basis.

Just over four years ago I was informed by a friend of a new technique developed by a reflexologist named Sally Kay. Apparently some trials had been undertaken with a few women who had developed lymphoedema. The trials had resulted in a reduction in the swelling of the affected limb. I was interested and keen to try this technique hoping this would improve my condition. I had heard of reflexology and the benefits to the body however had never actually tried it personally. I was aware reflexology involves pressure to the feet/hands and is viewed as alternative medicine. In December 2014 I contacted Sally Kay and made an appointment for my first treatment.

My arm at this point had become swollen, my hand and fingers were puffy and my shoulder ached. From the very first appointment I noticed a difference. The treatment itself is non-intrusive, it's relaxing and I certainly noticed a change. My arm was measured before the treatment commenced and then again after the therapy had been undertaken and sure enough there was a difference in the fluid. I continued the treatment for a number of weeks. By this time I felt my body was relaxed, my lymphatic system did not feel so sluggish and more importantly the swelling in my arm continued to drop. The reflexology session also helped release some tension and was beneficial in restoring balance and harmony in me which I had not felt for some time.

I have been attending reflexology sessions over the last four years, arranging appointments every five to six weeks. Initially there was a big reduction in the fluid loss, this has now wavered. However after each session there is still a change in the arm, although it may be slight it continues to decrease. I intend to continue with these sessions as I believe this technique in conjunction with the support of the lymphoedema compression garment is effective and beneficial in maintaining the fluid level in the affected limb.

I can only speak from a personal point of view and comment on my own individual experience of this treatment. For me as I reflect over the last few years I have found this treatment beneficial not only in helping reduce the swelling in my arm but also helping me relax and having a sense of wellbeing. I have also managed to lose weight and am now wearing jackets and cardigans comfortably.

Cancer or any association with the word cancer can be frightening and though cancer itself is not contagious the fear of it is. We live in a constantly changing world where medicine is advancing, research expanding, and progress evident in areas which once were deemed as impossible or untreatable. However the endurance and determination of individuals striving to make a difference and techniques such as this support and help alleviate the conditions of those affected by this disease.

2. Jan Rose, reflexologist – suitcase to clutch bag!

This is what my new client says about her lymphoedema

This client had breast cancer 10 years ago and had a mastectomy and 12 lymph nodes removed. In the years since then she has felt that she has been carrying a handbag between the arm on the affected side and her ribcage. It is not noticeably bigger than the other arm, but to her it feels like it. She has been telling her doctors this but says that "they looked at me as if I was crazy". Some days she says it felt like a suitcase. After just one session of RLD she says it has reduced to a clutch bag!

3. Ethne, research participant

In October 2004, I was diagnosed with breast cancer, and fortunate to be in the care of Mr. Simon Holt, Head of Department and Consultant Surgeon at the Prince Philip Hospital Breast Care Unit, Llanelli. After surgery, my tumour was diagnosed as Grade 3, and I received a course of chemotherapy followed by radiotherapy.

One of the side effects of breast cancer treatment is secondary lymphoedema, and I received treatment for this at the Lymphoedema Department at the hospital for over five years. I wore a compression sleeve on my affected arm during this time, until May 2012 when I was invited to attend the RLD research trial at the Princess of Wales Hospital, Bridgend.

The swelling in my affected arm improved remarkably over the trial, and I was able to cope very well without wearing my compression sleeve.

In those early days, there was no available RLD therapist in the Llanelli area or elsewhere in Carmarthenshire. After speaking to Mr. Simon Holt regarding the success of RLD and the problem of a local therapist, he agreed to sponsor Mrs. Susan Holcombe, a trained nurse and reflexologist in Llanelli, to attend a specialist training course on RLD given by Sally Kay. Susan now treats a number of patients suffering secondary lymphoedema in the Llanelli and Carmarthenshire area very successfully in their homes.

I will always be grateful to Sally Kay for developing such an effective therapy for the comfortable control of secondary lymphoedema, and wish her continued success in introducing RLD worldwide in the years ahead.

Many thanks Sally.

4. Reflexologist Rachael Posner's case study – "RLD is a game-changer."

I have been having reflexology treatments with various therapists for 20 years. However RLD treatment has been something of a game-changer and has proven particularly effective in helping to manage my long-term health conditions (ME and fibromyalgia). It is an energy-boosting treatment that has improved my overall wellbeing and flexibility and has also (I believe) been complementary to my current weight-loss programme. It is now my reflexology treatment of choice going forward and I would strongly recommend to others managing chronic health conditions or looking to lose weight. Sincere thanks to my wonderful therapist Rachael, who is highly skilled at putting this specialised treatment into practice with loving hands!

5. Dorothy Lawrie – primary lymphoedema

I just want to let you all know that the work that Sally Kay has done to design a routine specifically for lymphoedema has given you all the ability to have a positive effect on people's lives. I have primary lymphoedema, a condition I was born with and which I inherited from my mum. For years I knew how my future after 40 would go, as I watched my mum become less mobile every year as the lymph took over her life and her legs just got bigger and bigger. Each time she would go to see a medical professional, it was always classed as a weight problem. It was not until after she passed that I found out why she had "elephant legs" and that too was my future.

I feel myself lucky, it did not get bad for me until my forties, however there are children out there struggling daily, wondering why one leg is bigger than the other, why a small cut makes them ill if they get cellulitis and they cannot do what their friends do and that the heat makes the swelling worse.

I have trained in lymph massage, the Vodder technique, and yes it's fab. However it was time consuming, although a light massage it was right in your personal space and needed doing very, very regularly - and costly. Even on a fantastic salary it was expensive.

Life used to consist of getting out of bed wondering if I could leave the house today because I did not know if I could get shoes on, especially would I be able to finish a work outfit with acceptable shoes.

Imagine doing a presentation to a group of bankers in suits with crocs on, because nothing else fitted. I never wear skirts because I think people are staring at my fat feet coming over my shoes.

For a couple of years I followed Sally Kay's work intently and last year another wonderful person, Vicky Laws, took me on as a client and started doing RLD on me.

I am a therapist and always believe the intent to heal is there, however the results after the first session far, far exceeded my expectations.

Lymph almost immediately moved and started to exit my body.

Regular treatments have meant that my lymph is more manageable, and I can wear more normal shoes. I no longer get "heavy leg" syndrome in the evening.

I feel better, have not had sore throats that previously plagued me all winter and have even flown for the first time in years. I just made sure I did the hand routine frequently when away.

I have also realised that my condition had caused me social anxiety as I did not socialise or go to anything like the pictures for years. I gave up all that I loved doing. I would go out but on my own, head down and get on with it, so that my loved ones were not exposed to the stigma. I think that was only in my head though. I am great at outwardly appearing confident.

I just wanted to say a massive thanks to Sally Kay for her dedication to RLD, for giving life back to sufferers whether it is primary or secondary lymphoedema.

It is early days however, but I believe that my lymph system is getting stronger.

Sally has passed on this knowledge and I just wanted to give everyone a little insight into how this condition, although not life threatening, can be life impacting.

Thanks for reading.

Reflection

- A small sample of case studies and testimonials can underline the positive benefits of RLD
- Case studies provide valid anecdotal evidence
- Reflective practice is useful for personal and professional development

Chapter 11
The Full Circle

Back to the roots of reflexology

In 2016 I was lucky enough to visit China, surely the ultimate destination for a reflexologist. I was looking for inspiration to help with the final push to finish this book by going back to the ancient roots of reflexology to research, compare and contrast it with our practice in the UK. As part of the exploration I went for a reflexology/foot massage every day. In some places it is advertised as reflexology but mostly it is known as foot massage, but the difference was indiscernible.

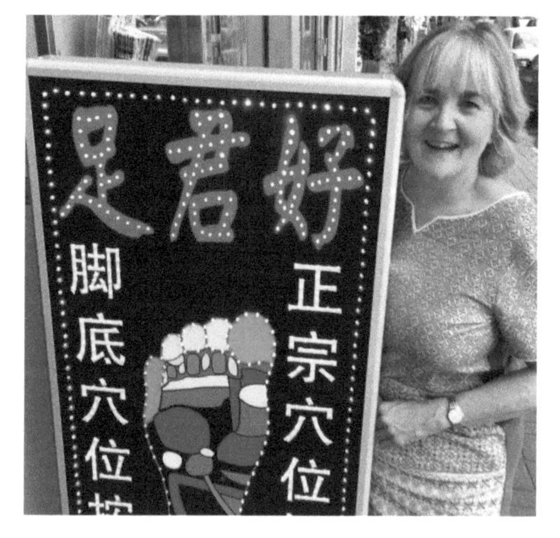

Fig. 40: **China, 16th July 2016**

It is commonplace to just walk in off the street without an appointment and be seen straight away. Many of the places are open all day and into the early hours of the morning. Although everywhere is different, the therapeutic experience is similar right across the board, whether it costs the equivalent of £5 or £50, day or night.

In every treatment I had, the pressure used was very deep, and sometimes painful. I did not experience any form of gentle treatment. Not much resembled UK reflexology practices. There was little variation in pressure, it was deep or deep and absolutely fascinating to watch each reflexologist work. They had such strong hands. I would find it difficult to work with this pressure all day.

Treatment always starts with a foot soak and sometimes a clothed acupressure style back, neck and shoulder massage while the feet are soaking. Other times acupressure massage is given after the feet have been worked on. When this happened after the reflexology, I suspected they were working on the areas of the body corresponding to the imbalances found on the feet. There was no way of knowing because of the language barrier, so communication was non-verbal only, and at no time was a consultation or medical history given.

Ruminating over this, I wondered if perhaps we pay too much attention and worry unnecessarily about contra-indications and cautions, although generally I think not. It was alright for me, as I did not have any known contra-indications.

Eagerly watching others receiving reflexology in the other chairs in the room, deep pressure was being applied all around and yet they did not seem to flinch like I did. This got easier the more I received. I understand it's commonplace for people to have this weekly.

Treatments were physical and very thorough and seemed to follow a similar sequence to that detailed here in Western reflexology foot map terms.

It began with a cup of flower tea and my feet were soaked in a deep wooden bucket full of hot water. When acupressure massage was given it started with my hands, arms, shoulder and upper lymph, along the clavicle, the occipital, neck and spine. It felt nice, in the kind of "good pain" sort of way, something reflexology clients say occasionally.

There were plenty of tender spots, possibly due to the recent long-haul flight to China. The reflexology began with my left foot, applying deep circular pressure to the spleen reflex with his knuckle. This followed with deep pressure from kidney to bladder reflexes with a knuckle, which was uncomfortable. Using the flat surface of his fist, the digestive and elimination reflexes were worked deeply in a clockwise direction, as you would expect. The treatment seemed to focus on circulation and elimination.

Next he worked along my toes, at the end of the meridians, then a fast vigorous sweep across the upper trapezius reflex, only working medial to lateral. The SCV reflex received a lot of attention, although pressure was much greater than that of RLD. This reflex was worked in a similar way, sliding down between the metatarsals (I am told this SCV reflex is Liver 3 acupressure point). The whole foot was manipulated, deeply and completely, until tender spots eased, before moving to the right foot, where the sequence began with the liver reflex, worked similarly using his knuckle.

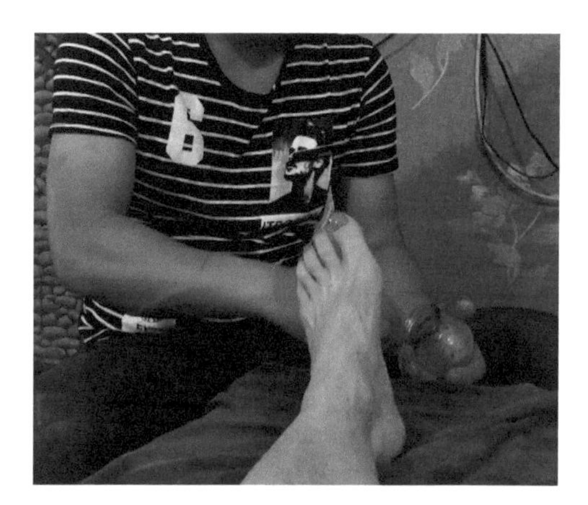

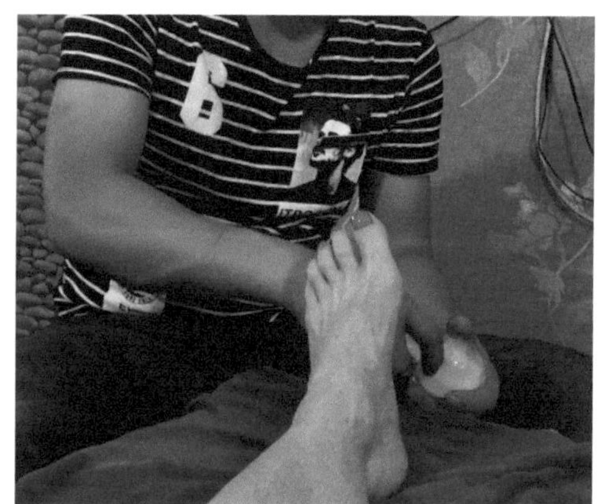

Fig. 41: **Cupping**

A few times I thought the treatment was over, with several false finishes. Both feet were wrapped in a lovely warm towel and he left the room. He returned with a small case containing glass cups, spray fuel and a lighter. Cupping on the plantar was a lovely move. The cup is sprayed with a flammable liquid, before being lit and placed over the sole of the foot. This creates a vacuum and the cup is used to massage the foot without breaking the suction. The kidney reflex on my right foot had been sensitive during the treatment. I could feel it again as the hot cup drew over the reflex, and it felt as if it was being drawn out of the sole of my foot as it dispersed. Each foot was wrapped in a towel with the cup still attached to the plantar abdominal reflexes. Again he left the room and I assumed that was it, but no. When he came back he removed the cups, and worked the lateral side of my leg. He used firm acupressure on the lower limb and tapotement (cupping with his hand) on the lateral side of my thigh. It was a noisy invigorating action. Again, I assumed this was the end, but finally he lifted each leg, one at a time, as high as it would go. It was a really good stretch to the lower back. I felt fantastic afterwards, thirsty but totally rejuvenated and energised.

Every session began with the left foot, which in my experience is the exception in the UK. They did however work each foot deeply and completely before moving on to the other foot, which I like very much. This is how I have always worked, and it's also the way I prefer to receive a reflexology treatment. I find it more fluent and relaxing than having the flow disrupted by swapping from one foot to the other, or worse still if both feet are worked simultaneously! Working 2 feet together does not work for me, without a supporting hand there is little resistance for different pressure on the reflexes. Instead both feet feel like they're flopping around rather than feeling held. It feels very odd, unsupported and unsatisfactory, maybe because I'm not used to it.

After working both feet separately, typically I would return to any reflexes, tender spots and areas of imbalance on the feet at the end of the treatment. Similarly in China areas of imbalance seem to be worked directly on the body rather than returning to the reflexes. Fascinating!

There was a lovely irony to spending time in China writing a book about a reflexology technique, developed in the UK, while enjoying as much Chinese reflexology as possible.

This experience was thought-provoking. Is there a right or wrong way? I genuinely do not believe there is, and instead prefer to stand by the principle of justifying applied therapeutic choices. The "why?" goes right back to Ted's biggest lesson. After all, he had spent years studying Chinese medicine in China, including reflexology foot massage. Being there was an insightful and inspirational experience, the full circle, right back to its ancient roots where it all began, ready to really start learning from the masters.

In reality, the reflexology we practise in the West has evolved into something quite different from that of the traditional Chinese foot massage reflexology. As we know it, reflexology is generally accepted as a relaxing experience, or just a placebo, depending who you ask, the premise being that everything else feels better in a relaxed state, as opposed to a tense or anxious one.

Either way we expect to feel a benefit after a treatment. This is true of my experience even though the therapeutic touch was different. Afterwards I felt fantastic, clear and totally energised!

As always, there are so many things to question and with this, the more I learn the less I know.

Chapter 12
The Future

Making waves with the ripple effect

What next and where do we go from here? We need to keep up the momentum, strengthen the evidence and help RLD to flow in the right direction. I believe that this treatment has the potential to be a sustainable, non-invasive solution to the management of breast cancer related lymphoedema.

The published studies alone (see Chapter 9 on page 167) do not provide enough evidence to prove conclusively the effect of RLD. However, the results are statistically significant enough to justify further research into the use of RLD in the management of breast cancer related lymphoedema.

There is a recurring theme in feedback from people receiving RLD, many feel similar sensations in the body during the treatment, including a "ripple", "waves", "a flow" as well as a cool sensation or a trickle as they feel the lymph begin to move. The more you work with RLD, you will begin to notice these responses as they happen during the sequence, often at the same time as certain reflexes are worked at the same stage in the treatment.

This repeated feedback has inspired senior reflexology lecturer at Cardiff Metropolitan University, Judith Whatley, to introduce thermal imaging technology to look at the movement and flow of lymph during RLD and reflexology. These thermal images (Figs. 44 & 45) are two (of many) that were taken during a pilot study.

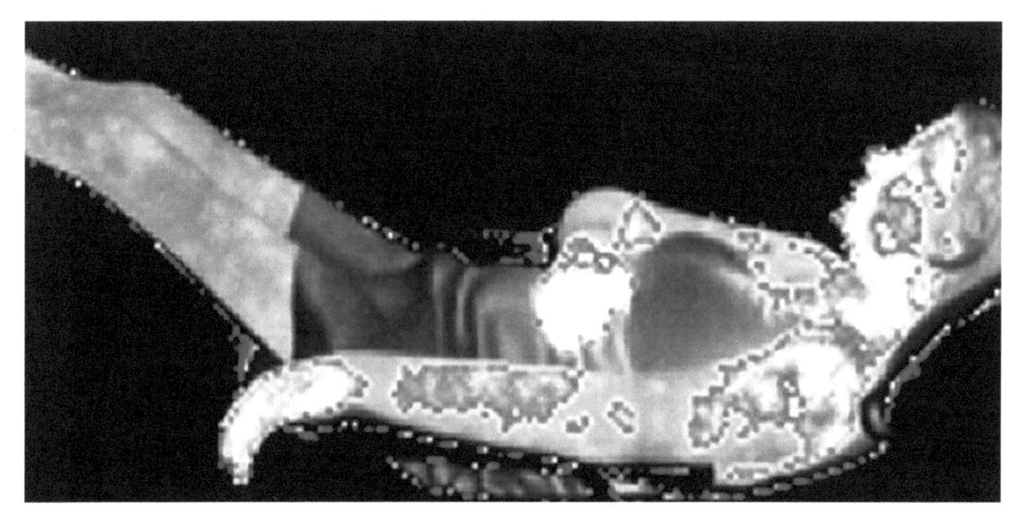

Fig. 42: **Thermal image taken as RLD began**

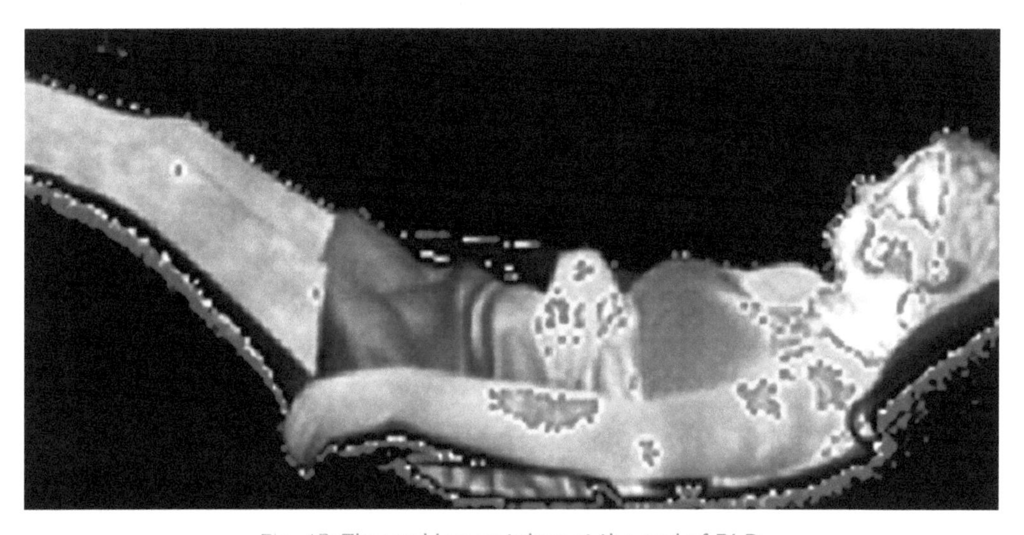

Fig. 43: **Thermal image taken at the end of RLD**

Cardiff Metropolitan University's School of Health Sciences aims to gradually expand this into a credible evidence base.

A dual crusade, making waves! The university can continue with further RLD research and the time and energy a PhD would have taken me has been put to a more practical use, writing this book, training other reflexologists and generally spreading the word. Subsequently many individuals are already experiencing the benefits of this adapted reflexology treatment. These include physical relief from the discomfort of lymphoedema swelling, and the psychological knock-on effect to the quality of life for breast cancer survivors. In addition to these well documented benefits, the surprise results have been a revelation, an added bonus to other people with all kinds of non-cancer related auto-immune disorders and inflammatory conditions, as previously seen in Chapter 2 on page 42, Chapter 9 on page 167 and Chapter 10 on page 186.

Will there come a time when complementary healthcare is truly mainstream? I do hope so, indeed the increasing recognition of the benefits of RLD by many healthcare professionals certainly supports this step in the right direction.

If you look back at the history of reflexology and other so-called wellbeing practices, such as yoga and meditation, massage or acupuncture, all of these modalities were used in ancient cultures to stay well and have been around for thousands of years. Sadly in the Western world people tend to turn to complementary and alternative therapies only when things go wrong.

Reflexology is a complementary therapy, not an alternative one, and as such it sits well alongside conventional medicine.

I believe that the ripple effects of RLD treatments will be seen in lymphoedema clinics throughout the UK, and ultimately worldwide when patients who have had RLD attend for their routine appointments and annual check-ups. I hope the ripple effect becomes a tidal wave of RLD and reflexology into a more integrated healthcare system. After all there is no magic pill for lymphoedema.

The health service is always looking for new and improved ways to treat patients. They are currently experimenting with Fluoroscopy Guided Manual Lymph Drainage (FG-MLD). This involves an invasive injection of indocyanine, fluorescent dye, into the limb for the problem to show up on the scan. I would imagine this is also a far more expensive intervention than RLD has the potential to be. Ultimately, a cost benefit analysis study to look into this would be ideal and the results may well influence decision making in the future.

RLD is a relaxing and enjoyable treatment. It has potential as a non-invasive, sustainable solution for the management of breast cancer related lymphoedema. I suspect it could also be a useful intervention to help those with other lymphatic disorders, such as primary lymphoedema and lipoedema.

It is heartwarming to have peer support and a shared goal working as a reflexologist. Together, we are a much stronger profession and more able to achieve a step change in our professional development and subsequent services.

Modern day attitudes to health and wellbeing mean that we never stop learning whilst keeping an open mind to other therapies and innovations. Being a reflexologist is not a competition! Sharing and collaboration is, I believe, the most effective way forward.

The journey continues with you...

Appendices

Step this way

Now that you have read this book, you understand the inception of RLD, its development, method and implementation.

I invite you to join and contribute to the momentum of this remarkable journey and stay connected for news and future developments. Together we can keep moving forward in the right direction, one small step at a time.

There is a DVD of the original RLD protocol and a foot chart which are available to order online at www.reflexologylymphdrainage.co.uk. This complements the book perfectly.

For more information about all things RLD related please go to the website www.reflexologylymphdrainage.co.uk where you will find details about RLD training courses for reflexology practitioners.

The website has links to social media.
Facebook group: Reflexology Lymph Drainage
Facebook page: Sally Kay Reflexology
Instagram: @sallyreflex
Twitter: @sallyreflex
YouTube: Sally Kay

These social medial platforms are great for easy access to extra hints and tips.

Useful sources of information

Books

Kane M. (2004). *Research Made Easy in Complementary and Alternative Medicine*, London: Churchill Livingstone

Mackereth P. and Carter A. (2006). *Massage & Bodywork: Adapting Therapies for Cancer Care*, London: Elselvier Limited

Mackereth P., Maycock P. and Tomlinson L. (2017) Easing the breathing body. In: Carter A. and Mackereth P. (Eds.) *Aromatherapy, Massage and Relaxation in Cancer Care: An Integrative Resource for Practitioners*, London: Jessica Kingsley Publications

Mortimer, Professor P. and Levine, G. (2017) *Let's Talk Lymphoedema, The Essential Guide to Everything You Need to Know*, London: Elliott & Thompson

Websites

British Lymphology Society (BLS)

The BLS is a dynamic and innovative body providing a strong professional voice and support for those involved in the care and treatment of people with lymphoedema and related lymphatic disorders, including lipoedema.

Website: www.thebls.com

Cancer Research UK

Cancer Research UK, Angel Building, 407 St John Street, London EC1V 4AD

Telephone: 020 7242 0200

Website: www.cancerresearchuk.org

Lymphoedema Support Network (LSN)

The Lymphoedema Support Network represents, supports and empowers people affected by lymphoedema, promotes awareness of the condition and campaigns for appropriate, equitable treatment for all.

Website: www.lymphoedema.org

Macmillan Cancer Support

89 Albert Embankment, London SE1 7UQ

Website: www.macmillan.org.uk

Measure Yourself Medical Outcome Profile (MYMOP) & Measure Yourself Concerns and Wellbeing (MYCaW)

Website: www.bris.ac.uk/primaryhealthcare/resources/mymop/

NHS

Website: www.nhs.uk

Tenovus Cancer Care

Head Office Tenovus Cancer Care, Gleider House, Ty Glas Road, Cardiff CF14 5BD

Telephone: 029 2076 8850

Website: www.tenovuscancercare.org.uk

Federation of Holistic Therapists (FHT)

18 Shakespeare Business Centre, Hathaway Close, Eastleigh SO50 4SR

Telephone: +44 (0)23 8062 4350

Email: info@fht.org.uk

Website: www.fht.org.uk

Association of Reflexologists

Victoria House, Victoria Street, Taunton, Somerset TA1 3FA

Email: info@aor.org.uk

Telephone: 01823 351010

Website: www.aor.org.uk

Glossary

BCRL Breast Cancer Related Lymphoedema

BLS British Lymphology Society

CAMSTRAND Complementary Alternative Medicine Strategy for Research and Development

CC Cisterna chyli

CPD Continuing Professional Development

CRUK Cancer Research UK

DLT Decongestive Lymphatic Therapy

LSN Lymphoedema Support Network

LVCM Limb Volume Circumference Measurements

MLD Manual Lymph Drainage massage

MLLB Multi-layer lymphoedema bandaging

MYCaW Measure Yourself Concerns and Wellbeing

MYMOP Measure Yourself Medical Outcome Profile

NACTHPC National Association of Complementary Therapists in Hospice and Palliative Care

RLD Reflexology Lymph Drainage

SCV Subclavian vein

SLD Simple Lymph Drainage self-help exercise/massage

VAS Visual Analogue Scale

Proximal - The nearest to the body or point of attachment

Distal - The furthest from the body or point of attachment

Medial - The nearest to the mid-line of the body

Lateral - The left & right side furthest from the mid-line of the body

Posterior - The back

Anterior - The front

Image Index

Charts

Chart 01: Percentage of excess swelling between the swollen arm & the normal arm on page 53

Participant 1:
Chart 02: Percentage difference between swollen & normal arm on page 168
Chart 03: Summary of the swollen arm on page 168
Chart 04: Proximal & distal ratio of swelling on page 169
Chart 05: MYCaW scores on page 169

Participant 2:
Chart 06: Percentage difference between swollen & normal arm on page 170
Chart 07: Summary of the swollen arm on page 170
Chart 08: Proximal & distal ratio of swelling on page 171
Chart 09: MYCaW scores on page 171

Participant 3:
Chart 10: Percentage difference between swollen & normal arm on page 172
Chart 11: Summary of swollen arm on page 172
Chart 12: Proximal & distal ratio of swelling on page 173
Chart 13: MYCaW scores on page 173

Participant 4:
Chart 14: Percentage difference between swollen & normal arm on page 174
Chart 15: Summary of the arm on page 174
Chart 16: Proximal & distal ratio of swelling on page 175
Chart 17: MYCaW scores on page 175

Participant 5:
Chart 18: Percentage difference between swollen & normal arm on page 176
Chart 19: Summary of swollen arm on page 176
Chart 20: Proximal & distal ratio of swelling on page 177
Chart 21: MYCaW scores on page 177

Participant 6:
Chart 22: Percentage difference between swollen & normal arm on page 178
Chart 23: Summary of swollen arm on page 178
Chart 24: Proximal & distal ratio of swelling on page 179
Chart 25: MYCaW scores on page 179

Images

Fig. 01: Anatomical reference for spine reflexes on page 20
Fig. 02: Atsitsa, August 2009 on page 27
Fig. 03: Hospice of the Valleys, February 2011 on page 33
Fig. 04: My graduation, July 2011 on page 34
Fig. 05: Poster presentation at CAMSTRAND, 29th March 2012 on page 35
Fig. 06: Before & After on page 56
Fig. 07: The lymphatic system and RLD on page 61
Fig. 08: Initial lymph capillary on page 62
Fig. 09: Lymph node on page 63
Fig. 10: Lymph nodes on page 63
Fig. 11: Cisterna chyli & thoracic duct on page 64
Fig. 12: Subclavian vein on page 64
Fig. 13: Right & left drainage on page 65
Fig. 14: Spleen on page 65
Fig. 15: Lateral view (Before & After) on page 74
Fig. 16: Posterior view (Before & After) on page 74
Fig. 17: Compression garment on page 80
Fig. 18: Bones of the feet on page 94

Fig. 19: Diaphragm on page 95
Fig. 20: Spine reflex on page 97
Fig. 21: Cisterna chyli & thoracic duct, subclavian vein on page 97
Fig. 22: Cisterna chyli reflex on page 99
Fig. 23: Thoracic duct on page 100
Fig. 24: Subclavian vein on page 102
Fig. 25: Cervical lymph nodes reflex on page 105
Fig. 26: Upper trapezius & back of underarm on page 105
Fig. 27: Upper lymph on page 110
Fig. 28: Lateral shoulder - deltoid reflex on page 114
Fig. 29: Upper lymph to underarm reflexes on page 118
Fig. 30: Lower lymphatic reflexes (medial to lateral) on page 122
Fig. 31: Lower lymph (lateral to medial) thoracic duct & subclavian vein on page 122
Fig. 32: Breast reflex on page 128
Fig. 33: Arm reflex on page 131
Fig. 34: Spleen on page 136
Fig. 35: Kidney to bladder reflex on page 137
Fig. 36: Hand reflexes for RLD on page 142
Fig. 37: Upper lymph hand reflexes on page 142
Fig. 38: 4cm cylinders of the arm on page 159
Fig. 39: Lymphoedema measurement sheet on page 208
Fig. 40: China, 16th July 2016 on page 216
Fig. 41: Cupping on page 218
Fig. 42: Thermal image taken as RLD began on page 222
Fig. 43: Thermal image taken at the end of RLD on page 222

Tables

Table 1: Baseline MYCaW concerns on page 49
Table 2: Summary on page 50

Index

Symbols

4cm cylinder 159

A

Abdominal organs 64
Accidents 69
Acupressure 217
Acupuncture 223
Adapt the treatment 143
Afferent lymph vessels 62
Ancient roots of reflexology 216
Antibodies 66
Antigens 63, 65
Anxiety 149, 151
Arm 131
Arm reflex 131
Arterial oxygenated blood 60
Association of Reflexologists 39
Auto-immune conditions 143, 145
Auto-immune disorders 223
Axilla reflex 110
Axillary lymph nodes 118

B

Back of the underarm 74, 107
Bacteria 66
Bacterial 78
Bandaging 79
Bandaging treatment 209
Bartholin's cyst case study 196
Baseline 47
Baseline summary 50
Bicuspid valves 62
Bilateral 144
Bilateral secondary lymphoedema of the arms 144
Bladder 137, 139
Blood capillaries 60
Blood circulation 63
Blood plasma 60
Bone marrow 66
Breast cancer related lymphoedema 72, 188
Breast cancer related lymphoedema case study 205, 207
Breast cancer related lymphoedema of the arm case study 198
Breast reflex 128
British Lymphology Society 84

C

CAM 35
CAMSTRAND 35
Cancer Research UK 72, 73
Capillaries 62
Casley-Smith 84
Cautions 148
Cellular debris 60, 63, 65
Cellulitis 78, 152
Cervical lymph nodes 105
Cervical lymph nodes reflex 106
Chemotherapy 72, 209
Chemotherapy cycle 72
Chemotherapy wards 150
China 91, 216
Chinese foot massage reflexology 220
Chronic fatigue syndrome 145
Cisterna chyli 64, 99
Cisterna chyli reflex 99, 125
Cleaning windows 79
Clinical experience 25
Clinical reasoning 149
Collaboration 224
Complex medical health problems 151
Compression 76
Compression garment 74, 80
Compression garments 79
Conceptual framework 47
Consent 47
Constipation 26, 28
Consultation 47
Contra-indications 148, 149
Contra-indications for RLD 152
Conventional medicine 223
Cost benefit analysis 224
Critical thinking 148
Cuneiform bone 64, 99
Cupping 218
Cycling 79
Cylinder of the arm 159
Cytotoxic drugs 72

D

Damaged red blood cells 65
Dame Cicely Saunders 22
Decongestive Lymphatic Therapy 76
Deep vein thrombosis 152
Deltoid 114
Deltoid muscle reflex 114
De-oxygenated blood 60
Diagnosis 151
Diaphragm reflex 95
Domiciliary visits 24
Dorsal 110
Drainage action 66
Drop-in clinics 28
Dusting 79

E

Efferent lymph vessels 63
Emotional distress 151
Empty space 93
End of life organ failure 152
Everyday living activities 70
Exercise 76, 79

F

Fatty acids 60
Fear 70, 149
Feathering 139
Federation of Holistic Therapists 39
FG-MLD 224
Fibromyalgia 145
First principles of RLD 92
Flow 139
Fluid under the arm 73
Fluorescent dye 224
Fluoroscopy Guided Manual Lymph Drainage 224
Fluttering 30
Földi 84
Foot soak 217
Formula 163
Full sleeve 79
Fungal 78

G

Glove 79
Gravity 60
Guilt 149

H

Half sleeve 79
Headache 29
Health related worries 149
Hereditary 68
Home help tip 142
Home visits 150
Hospice of the Valleys 22, 24, 26, 35

I

Ileum 66
Immune response 66
Indocyanine 224
Infections 78
Inflammatory, auto-immune disorders 145
Initial lymphatics 62
Initial lymph capillaries 62
Injury 69
Insect bites 69
Integrating RLD 143

Interstitial spaces 60, 62
Intestinal wall 66
Intestine 64
Ironing 79

K

Kidney 137
Kidney to bladder 137
Kidney to bladder reflexes 137

L

Large lymphatic pathways 63
Larger lymph vessels 63
Largest lymphatic vessel 64
Lateral shoulder 114
Leduc 84
Left arm 83, 93
Left lymphatic duct 65
Left subclavian vein 65
Legs 64
Life limiting conditions 149
Lifetime risk 69, 72
Light feathering 30
Light pins and needles 139
Limb Volume Circumference Measurement 158
Linking 138
Lipoedema 145, 224
Lower limb swelling case study 201
Lower lymph 122
Lower lymph reflexes 123
LVCM 48, 158
Lymph 62
Lymphatic ducts 62
Lymph journey 62, 92
Lymph node 63
Lymph nodes 63
Lymphocytes 63, 66
Lymphoedema 68
Lymphoedema clinic 80
Lymphoedema clinics 223
Lymphoedema of the left arm 93
Lymphoedema of the right arm 93
Lymphoedema Support Network 77, 84
Lymphoedema swelling of the legs 144
Lymph vessels 62

M

Macmillan 73
Macrophages 63
Manual Lymph Drainage 76, 82
Massage 223
Mathematical formula 163, 164
Measure Yourself Medical Concerns and Wellbeing (MYCaW) 44
Measure Yourself Medical Outcome Profile (MYMOP) 44
Meditation 223

Meridians 218
Metatarsal 64
MLD 82, 91
MLLB 82
Movement 60
Multi-layer lymphoedema bandaging 82
Muscle pump effect 79
Muscular movement 60
MYCaW 47, 54

N

NACTHPC 36
Natural drainage 82
Nausea 26
Navicular 99
Neck reflex 106
NHS ethics 33, 91
Non-invasive 221, 224

O

Oedema 152
One-way drainage 60
One-way valve 62
Oral cavity 66
Original protocol 91

P

Pain 26
Palliative care 150
Palliative case study 192
Particulate waste 60
Pathogens 60, 63, 65
Pathology of the disease 151
Peer support 24
Peyer's patches 66
Phagocytosis 63, 65
Pharynx 66
Pilates 79
Pins and needles 30
Placebo 220
Plasma 60
Power of suggestion 145
Presenting conditions 148
Prevention 77
Primary lymphoedema 68, 145, 213, 224
Professional development 224
Prognosis 151
Protein-rich interstitial fluid 69
Proteins 60
Psoriatic arthritis case study 199
Psychological peristalsis 143
Psychological side effects 70
Pulmonary embolism 152

Q

Quality of life 70

R

Radiation 69
Radiotherapy 72
Recovery 70
Reflexology client groups 149
Research abstract 167
Research case studies 167
Reservoir 64
Right arm 83, 93
Right lymphatic duct 65
Right subclavian vein 65
Ripple 30
Rippling 139

S

Safe practice 25, 148, 150
Scan 224
Scapula reflex 107
Scar tissue 69
Secondary lymphoedema 69
Secondary lymphoedema, post-operative inflammation and pain case study 194
Self-care 77
Self-confidence 70
Sensations 139
Side effects 148
Simple data collection 44
Simple Lymph Drainage 84, 85
Skin care 76, 78
SLD 84, 91
Sleeplessness 26
Soft tissue 62
Solution to the management of breast cancer related lymphoedema 221
Spinal cord 98
Spinal cord reflex 98
Spleen 65
Spleen reflex 136
Stage of the disease 151
Subclavian vein 62, 63, 102, 110
Subclavian vein reflex 100, 102, 107
Subjective 54
Superficial initial lymph 62
Supervision 24
Surgery 69
Survivorship 70
Sustainable 221
Sustainable solution 224
Swimming 79
Symptoms 148, 151
Symptoms of lymphoedema 70

T

Tenovus 55
Thermal imaging 221
Thoracic duct 64
Thoracic duct reflex 99, 125
Thymus 66
Tingling 30, 139
T lymphocytes 66
Tonsils 66
Transport 60
Trauma 69
Trickle 139

U

Underarm 105, 107, 118
Undiagnosed swelling 152
Unstable heart conditions 152
Upper lymph 110
Upper lymph reflexes 110
Upper trapezius 105, 107
Upper trapezius reflex 107
Urination 30

V

Vacuuming 79
Viral 78
Visual Analogue Scale (VAS) 44
Vodder 84
Volume 163

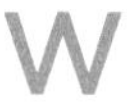

W

Walking 79
Wave 30, 139
Weakness 70
Welsh cancer charity 55

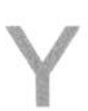

Y

Yoga 79, 223